nas

Medical Nur

CW00555281

nas

nas

Medical Nursing
A Concise Nursing Text

Gillian M. Newton SRN, DN(Lond)
Ward Sister, The London Hospital, Whitechapel

Clive Andrewes SRN, RMN, DN(Lond), BSc
Charge Nurse, The London Hospital, Whitechapel

Tenth Edition

Baillière Tindall London Philadelphia Toronto
Mexico City Rio de Janeiro Sydney Tokyo Hong Kong

Baillière Tindall
———————
W.B. Saunders

1 St Anne's Road
Eastbourne, East Sussex BN21 3UN, England

West Washington Square
Philadelphia, PA 19105, USA

1 Goldthorne Avenue
Toronto, Ontario M8Z 5T9, Canada

Apartado 26370—Cedro 512
Mexico 4, DF Mexico

Rua Evaristo da Veiga, 55,20° andar
Rio de Janeiro–RJ, Brazil

ABP Australia Ltd, 44–50 Waterloo Road
North Ryde, NSW 2113, Australia

Ichibancho Central Building, 22–1 Ichibancho
Chiyoda-ku, Tokyo 102, Japan

10/fl, Inter-Continental Plaza, 94 Granville Road
Tsim Sha Tsui East, Kowloon, Hong Kong

First published 1941
Ninth edition 1977
Tenth edition 1984
Spanish translation, eighth edition (CECSA, Mexico)
Portuguese translation, eighth edition (Publicacoes Europa–America, Mira–Sintra)
Turkish edition (Turkish Government)

Margaret Hitch wrote the first edition of *Medical Nursing* and subsequent editions were prepared by Marjorie Houghton, the seventh in collaboration with Mary Whittow. The eighth and ninth were prepared by Christine M. Chapman. The tenth edition was written by Gillian M. Newton and Clive Andrewes.

Typeset by Herts Typesetting Services Ltd., Hertford
Printed and bound in Great Britain by
William Clowes Ltd., Beccles and London.

British Library Cataloguing in Publication Data

Newton, Gillian M.
 Medical nursing.–10th ed.–(Nurses' aids series)
 1. Nursing
 I. Title   II. Andrewes, Clive
 III. Chapman, Christine M. Medical nursing
 IV. Series   610.73 RT41

ISBN 0 7020 0963 6

Contents

Foreword

Medical Nursing in the Nurses' Aids Series, first published in 1941, is a book which has proved its worth over many years. One of its strengths has been the way in which it has not only kept up to date in medical terms, but has reflected changes in the way in which nurses have perceived and performed their role.

This is true of this new edition, written by two new authors, one a ward sister and the other a charge nurse. They have reflected the change in the delivery of nursing care by focusing on the 'problem identification approach' as demonstrated in the nursing process.

This is a handy (literally), concise reference book, which forms the basis of the information nurses require about medical nursing and, as such, should make an invaluable contribution to the personal library of the nurse learner. I wish it well.

C.M. Chapman, OBE Professor of Nursing Education
The Welsh National School of Medicine
Cardiff, Wales

Preface

Man, unlike any other thing organic or inorganic in the universe, grows beyond his work, walks up the stairs his concepts, emerges ahead of his accomplishments.

John E. Steinbeck from *The Grapes of Wrath*

It is now seven years since *Medical Nursing* was revised by Christine Chapman. In those years, nursing has experienced many changes, including those directed towards individualized nursing care.

In rewriting this book we have applied a problem-solving approach to the care of patients. We have included new chapters on the care of the dying and on people in hospital, which covers individualized patient care, psychological aspects of care and discharge planning.

Christine Chapman has stated previously that a book of this size must be selective. This remains true. Specialized chapters such as infectious diseases have been reduced and we have omitted the chapter on psychiatric disorders. We have identified the key points of nursing care in discussing common medical conditions. We hope this book will provide the basic information to carry out nursing care with understanding, and that it will stimulate nurses to explore their subject more deeply.

Gillian M. Newton
Clive Andrewes

Acknowledgements

For our students,
who provided the inspiration and motivation.

We are deeply indebted to our colleagues at The London Hospital for their help and encouragement with this book. Special thanks are due to Denise Barnett.

Kevin Marks worked with us closely on the artwork to illustrate the text with such clarity. We would also like to thank the London Hospital for their permission to use the nursing assessment form, the care plan form and the pain chart.

We are very grateful to Rosemary Long, Nursing Editor of Baillière Tindall, for her friendly guidance and interest, and for her patience.

Many thanks to Alison Cartmale and Sally Hounsell for their efficient typing.

Finally we must thank our friends for tolerating the long silences and periods of irritability.

1
People in Hospital

Admission to hospital is a stressful experience. The person facing admission is beset by anxiety over his health and concerned about the environment he is entering. These worries become more complex as he is transformed by the admission procedure from a person into a patient. His life outside hospital and his individuality and personality diminish as he assumes his role in the organizational structure. Nurses have a vital role to play in ensuring that people retain their individuality in hospital.

This chapter will consider:

- The admission procedure
- Individual nursing care (the 'nursing process')
- Psychological care
- Discharge from hospital

Admission to hospital

People are normally admitted in a planned way from home or as an emergency through the casualty department. This section will focus on the planned admission, although most of the comments are also relevant to an emergency admission.

People enter a ward dressed in their own clothes. They may be accompanied by relatives or friends, who are often asked to wait outside the ward. They are taken to their beds, the curtains are drawn, and they are asked to undress. They put on their nightwear, place their clothes in a locker, and get into bed. An identity band is placed around their wrist. They now have a number. Their family say goodbye and go home. They have now become patients in numbered beds.

In many cases this transformation need not be so rapid or bleak. The admission procedure should be organized so as to lessen the process of dehumanization and help a person retain his individuality. There are a number of ways this can be done:

- There is often little point in undressing quickly, as the doctor's examination may not take place for several hours. There may be no reason why people should not wear their own clothes for the greater part of their admission.
- People and their families should be warmly welcomed to the ward and shown where the day room and lavatories are. The different grades of nurses should be explained. A hot drink can be offered, as they may have travelled some distance or had a long wait before coming to the ward.
- Tasks, such as obtaining a urine specimen, taking the temperature or weighing, should not be done immediately, as people may feel these are more important than conversation.
- Where possible, admission should be calm, friendly and unhurried. Anxiety should be reduced by providing information and conveying the message that the person himself is important.

An interesting question is the extent to which it will benefit the person and the nurse to create a 'patient role'. When roles are well established, both nurse and patient know their place and may feel secure and safe. The creation of such a structured relationship may make it easier to give physical nursing care. However, the cost may be that psychological fears and anxiety are suppressed and, as a result, recovery may be delayed.

Nurses should care for the person as a whole. If individuality is reduced, this function cannot be fulfilled. The person will become simply 'the patient in bed ten with bronchitis'. Therefore, the admission procedure must be carried out in a way that prevents this occurring.

Once a person has been admitted it is necessary for him to maintain his independence and individuality. This can best be done by organizing nursing care on the basis of the individual's needs and problems. One of the ways of achieving this is through the use of the nursing process.

The nursing process

The nursing process is a problem-orientated approach designed to give individual nursing care. It is an attempt to organize nursing on the basis of the individual's own needs and problems. He is viewed against the background of his environment, his feelings about his health, and his attitude to his illness.

There are a number of concepts and theoretical models underlying the nursing process; these can be explored further by consulting the literature in the Further Reading list.

There are four stages to the nursing process:
● Assessment
● Planning
● Implementation
● Evaluation

Therefore a nurse assesses a person's problems, organizes her care to meet that problem, gives that care, and then reviews whether or not it has helped. These stages do not always occur in sequence; they can overlap each other and should be regarded as a continuous process.

Assessment
In order to plan individual nursing care it is necessary to assess the person's needs. There are a number of sources of information:

● The person himself
● His family
● Physical examination
● Medical case notes

Information about the person is often obtained using a systematic questionnaire. There are a number of different forms in use, each of them designed to provide information on:

● The person's current health and past medical history
● Social information — family, housing, occupation, etc.
● The person's level of independence — what he can or cannot do for himself
● The person's description of his normal daily living activities — sleep pattern, diet, elimination, etc.
● The person's senses — hearing, vision, etc. — described by the nurse in conjunction with the person.
● The person's response to his illness and admission to hospital

An example of a nursing assessment form is shown in Figure 1.

The questionnaire has a number of benefits in addition to the information it provides:

NURSING ADMISSION SHEET   ADULT PATIENTS

*Record Number _____
PATIENT LABEL
*Consultant _____
*House Officer _____
*Name _____
*Address _____
*Diagnosis _____
_____

*Date of birth _____ *Age _____
*Date of admission _____ *Time _____
*Type: Emergency   Waiting List
Transfer from _____
*Operations on present admission/
date performed: _____
_____
*Marital status _____ *Religion _____
*Next of kin (name) _____
*Relationship to patient _____
*Address _____
*Past medical history/operations _____
_____
_____

*Tel. no(s). _____
*Allergies _____
Speech difficulty/language barrier _____
*History of present complaint _____

CARE AT HOME   Details/Names
Community Nurse _____
*Other current health problems _____

Social Worker _____

Social Services (specify) _____
*What patient says is the reason for
admission _____
_____

*G.P. (name) _____
*Address _____

NURSING REMINDERS _____
_____
_____

SOCIAL HISTORY   Occupation _____
Children _____
Other dependants _____
HOUSING (house, flat — which floor,
stairs, lives alone, shares,
bathroom/toilet) _____
_____

Other problems at home? _____

Visiting problems?   Yes   No
If Yes, describe _____
DISCHARGE PLANNING — Please tick
those required, add date when
ordered or done.
                              Date
                    Needed   ordered

Social Services
(specify) _____

Community Nurse _____
*TTA's and Teaching _____
*Out-patient's appt. _____
*Transport _____
*Relatives informed _____

DAILY LIVING

DIET
*Special
Food or drink dislikes

Appetite: Good Poor
Remarks

SLEEP How many hours usually?
Sedation
Other comments
ELIMINATION
BOWELS Any problems: Yes No
If Yes, describe

How often are bowels opened?

Any medication?
URINARY No problems Incontinence
  Nocturia Dysuria
  Frequency Urgency
Remarks

FEMALE PATIENTS—MENSTRUATION
  Regular Irregular
  Amenorrhoea Dysmenorrhoea
  Post-menopausal Taking the Pill
Next period due
Will need: ST's Tampons
Remarks

HEARING Right: Good Poor Deaf
  Left: Good Poor Deaf
Hearing Aid? Yes No
Remarks
VISION Right: Good Poor Blind
  Left: Good Poor Blind
  Glasses Contact lenses
Remarks
PROSTHESES/APPLIANCES/AIDS
Type(s)

Any help needed? No Yes
MOBILITY Fully mobile? Yes No
If No, needs help with:
  Walking Standing Dressing
  Washing Bathing Feeding
  In/out of bed In/out of chair
Other (describe)

ORAL
Any problems with mouth or teeth?
  Yes No
If Yes, describe
Wears dentures?
  No Yes: Upper Lower
Any problems with dentures?

Any crowns?
SMOKING HABITS Non-smoker
Smokes: pipe cigars cigarettes

NURSE'S OBSERVATIONS

*ATTITUDE
  Anxious Withdrawn Distressed
Remarks (If particular problem please
try and state reason, e.g. anxious about
operation/or being in hospital, etc.)

GENERAL APPEARANCE
  Normal Obese
  Dehydrated Thin
  Acutely ill Emaciated
Remarks

SKIN
  Satisfactory Broken areas
  Dehydrated Rash
  Oedematous Jaundiced
Describe

LEVEL OF CONSCIOUSNESS
  Orientated Semi-conscious
  Confused Unconscious
Remarks

NORTON SCORE:

Information obtained: From   By   Level of training/position   Date   Time

Figure 1. Example of a nursing assessment form.

- It begins the relationship between the nurse and the person who is ill
- It strengthens the nurse's perception of the person as an individual
- It helps the person to realize he will be treated as an individual

It is important to explain to the person, before starting the questionnaire, that the information is being obtained in order to plan his individual nursing care. Questions should be asked quietly, as the information is personal and private. The person should not be made to feel he is discussing his affairs with the whole ward.

Assessment is *not* a rigid routine to be carried out at a particular time; it is a continuous activity. In an emergency admission, the type and degree of assessment will be, of course, appropriate to the particular circumstances.

Planning

Once an assessment has been made of the person's problems, a plan of care is drawn up. An example of a care plan form is given in Figure 2.

The problems identified will be seen from the perspective of the person or the nurse. Only those problems needing nursing care should be stated. Where possible, the reasons for the problem should be given. Problems should be listed in order of importance. However, this is not always possible, as priorities may change.

Where practicable, the person should be involved in planning his own care, since the aims of the nursing care are written from his point of view. It is necessary to include his opinion or the goals may be unrealistic.

Goals/aims

Having identified the problems, the next step is to decide on the nursing care required. A goal or aim is stated for each problem, and a time set for the review or evaluation of each.

Setting goals is often the area that causes most difficulty. If nursing care is to be reviewed accurately, goals must be specific. It is of little help if a goal is too general, e.g. 'not to be breathless'. A better goal would be 'not to be breathless while sitting in a chair or walking to the lavatory'. It is then possible to measure or evaluate whether the goal has been reached.

NURSING CARE PLAN

Name _____

Date	Patient's Problems	Goals/Outcome	NURSING ACTION				
			Date	Date	Date	Date	Date
		A					
		Review: Evaluation:					
		B					
		Review: Evaluation:					
		C					
		Review: Evaluation:					
		D					
		Review: Evaluation:					
		E					
		Review: Evaluation:					

Figure 2. Example of a care plan form.

Nursing instructions. Confusion will exist among nurses unless instructions are specific. 'Encourage fluids' or 'gradual mobilization' are two examples of general instructions which are open to a variety of interpretations. Communication between nurses is more effective if instructions are specific, e.g. 'to have 2500 ml of fluid over 24 hours (08.00–14.00, 800 ml; 14.00–22.00, 1200 ml; 22.00–08.00, 500 ml). Instructions should be precise and understood in the same way by every nurse involved in caring for that person.

Implementation

'Implementation' means giving the care that has been planned. The writing down of the plans does not automatically mean that they will be carried out. The plans for care must be communicated to the nurse (or nurses) involved, who must decide when to carry out the care, and then give it.

The use of this approach relies upon a system of allocating patients to nurses. It will not work if nurses are allocated tasks to perform rather than a particular group of people to nurse.

There will be times when staffing levels make it difficult to carry out this approach. This does not mean the approach is wrong, but rather that too few nurses are being employed to give adequate care. Documentation of such incidents may make it possible to examine scientifically how many nurses, at which grades, are actually needed.

The nursing care given is recorded in the progress notes/Kardex. An example of a progress form is given in Figure 3. It is important to record comments in relation to the problems in the care plan. For example, it is not the fact that a dressing has been performed that is relevant, but the condition of the wound. Similarly, it is not the fact that certain observations have been recorded every half an hour that is important, but rather the condition of the person.

Evaluation

In order to determine if nursing care is effective, it has to be evaluated. This is a continuous process which is difficult, or impossible, unless goals are stated in a way that can be measured.

DATE	TIME (24 hour clock)	PROGRESS NOTES	NURSE (Signature)
WARD:		BED NO: NAME:	

Figure 3. Example of a progress form.

Dates or times for reviewing each problem are included in the original care plan. At these times the nurse assesses whether the aim has been achieved. If it has not, either the nursing care or the goal must be altered.

Evaluation is important for the nursing profession. It provides the information that enables nurses to assess the effectiveness of their care. Nursing interventions which fail can be discarded and new approaches devised. Different approaches to the same nursing problem can be evaluated. A body of written information is thus being collected that enables nurses themselves to monitor and assess nursing actions.

General comments

The nursing process remains a subject of discussion and debate in nursing. It is important to remember that it is an *approach* to nursing care. It has within it the flexibility to adapt to the particular needs and illnesses of individuals. Involving the person in planning his care strengthens his role as an individual, rather than a passive, dependent patient. Such an approach fits in well with Virginia Henderson's famous definition of nursing found in *Basic Principles of Nursing Care* (published by the International Council of Nurses, London, in 1960):

'Nursing is primarily assisting the individual (sick or well) in the performance of those activities contributing to health, or its recovery (or to a peaceful death) that he would perform unaided if he had the necessary strength, will or knowledge. It is likewise the unique contribution of nursing to help the individual to be independent of such assistance as soon as possible.'

Psychological care

A person admitted to a general hospital will cope with the stress in the same way as he copes with other stresses in his life. He will have learnt ways to buffer himself against anxiety and external dangers. These 'defence mechanisms' — repression, reaction formation, rationalization, insulation and projection — are designed for self-protection, and they enable us to cope with our environment.

In hospital, a person is subjected to great stress. His ability to cope with anxiety will be tested to its limits. Not only is he concerned in a general way about his illness, his family and his new environment, but he is also subject to a range of specific anxieties over tests, operations and other aspects of hospital life.

Nurses are concerned with both the physical and psychological needs of people. These needs are inter-related; a person cannot be split into physical and emotional categories. Nurses must be constantly aware of an individual's psychological needs — such needs are not an extra part of the care to be met if there is enough time.

The main way of giving psychological care is through communication. Communication is essential for the establishment and maintenance of human relationships. It is the way people in hospital obtain information about their illness, tell nurses their problems, keep in contact with their families, and relate to other people on the ward. Communication can be verbal or non-verbal, or, as it is sometimes expressed, talking with or without words.

Verbal communication

Use of language involves the skills of:

- Speaking
- Listening
- Reading and writing

Speaking not only involves what is said, but how it is said. Messages about feeling are conveyed by the tone and inflection of the voice. 'Would you like another cup of tea?' can be asked in a friendly, positive way or in a grudging, negative manner.

When information is given, it should be precise and free of nursing or medical jargon. It is often helpful if the nurse asks the person to report back, in his own words, what she has said. This ensures he understands what was meant by her explanation.

In our multi-racial society some people may not speak English. In this case, a relative or interpreter can be used to convey information to them, and non-verbal communication assumes great importance.

Listening is an active process; it is much more than just hearing. It involves sharing information and feelings. Encouraging the person to express himself will not be helped if the person senses you are not listening. It means being attentive, not being silent.

Reading and writing are skills which are often taken for granted. There are, however, a large number of people who are unable to perform these skills and to assume that they can may cause distress and embarrassment.

Non-verbal communication / talking without words

Non-verbal communication can be the most effective means a nurse has of allaying fears and anxieties. It is a two-way method of communication that involves our five senses. Actions are transmitted as clearly as the spoken word, and they are understood as readily. Some actions communicate messages; others convey information about feelings or personality.

Body language. Gestures, movements of the body, facial expressions and posture all communicate messages. The way one approaches a person is vital in establishing a relationship. A smile, eye contact and an open posture, suggest friendliness and interest. The posture of a person who is huddled up in bed, with his back to the nurse, suggests withdrawal, apathy or depression. An illustration of how body language can convey information is shown in Figure 4.

A nurse needs to be aware of the messages being given by her own body, and those being sent by the individual in hospital.

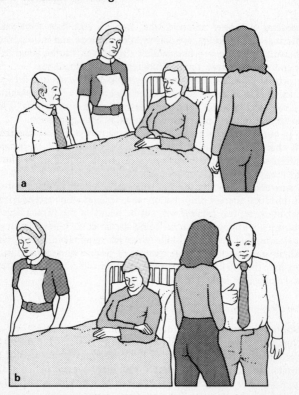

Figure 4. Examples of (a) good communication, and (b) poor communication using body language.

Touch. In nursing, touch may be the most important of all non-verbal behaviours. It is the most personal of our senses as it brings two human beings into a direct relationship. It is through touch that we feel the emotions of others. It is clearly a very powerful method of communication.

People are touched by nurses continually. It is an integral part of most nursing procedures. How the nurse handles or touches a person says a great deal about the way she feels about him and his illness. Similarly, touch tells the nurse a lot about a person's physical and emotional condition. Resting a hand on someone's shoulder, or holding their hand, can provide more emotional support than any number of words. Recognition of the importance of touch has perhaps diminished in modern medicine and nursing. However, its role should always be remembered.

Other aspects of non-verbal communication include periods of silence, the concept of territory, time, and vocalization (i.e., all aspects of sound — pitch, tone, screams, gasps, sighs, etc.).

Anxiety and stress are part of a person's life in hospital. Through verbal and non-verbal communication, the nurse must understand and meet the psychological needs of the people she is nursing. Therefore an understanding of the methods of communication is essential, or fears and worries will be ignored. Instead of nursing the person, as a whole, only the physical problems will be cared for.

Meeting a person's psychological needs in a constructive way will help him not only during his period in hospital, but will also enable him to re-enter his environment outside hospital more easily.

Discharge from hospital

Discharge from hospital is usually seen as a pleasant event. However, for some people it can be accompanied by stress. Many people are discharged on the same day as they are told they can go home. Anxieties can arise about the journey home, coping on arriving there, and the sudden change of environment. In addition, there are worries over drugs, possible dietary restrictions, and what activities should or should not be carried out.

The nurse has an important role in planning the person's discharge so as to ease these concerns. She acts as a co-ordinator of the people who are to give advice and arrange help in the community.

Throughout a person's stay in hospital, care should be given while bearing in mind the person's family and home environment. He should not be nursed solely within the framework of the hospital. The assessment of the person on admission and during his stay in hospital should reveal needs associated with the home situation. There are a number of factors of particular importance.

Need for understanding about the illness and its consequences

Advice and understanding about a person's illness is often necessary for the individual and his family, if his health is to be maintained.

- Knowledge about drugs regularly required and their side-effects is essential. Where possible, people should have their own drugs before discharge. They are then able to take them under supervision, and can familiarize themselves with when to take them and in what doses.

- Advice about diet may be required. The dietician should see the person and his family before discharge and, if possible, a person should choose his own diet on the ward. It is of little benefit if his diet is given to him the moment before he goes home, as he will have had no practice at choosing the correct foods.

- Information about the range and extent of activities which can be undertaken is often required. There may be restrictions on the amount of exercise, and on when to return to work or to resume sexual relationships. There are explanatory leaflets on many diseases which may be helpful, e.g. *A Heart Attack*, which is one of a series of booklets published by the British Heart Foundation.

- Information about the disease itself may be necessary. A person may need to recognize when he is having a hypo- or hyperglycaemic attack, or may need to know what to do if he is getting chest pain.

Ability to be independent

A person's ability to manage when he goes home must be considered in advance of his discharge. There are a number of services and aids which can be of help.

- A person may have nursing needs when at home. He may be unable to give his own insulin injection, or may need a nurse to perform a wound dressing. Community nurses can be arranged to help with such problems.

- He may be unable to shop, cook or look after his own house, and thus home helps or meals-on-wheels may need to be arranged.

● A home assessment by the occupational therapist and social worker may be undertaken. If required, practical aids such as a commode, rails in the bathroom, or a different bed can be arranged.

Living accommodation

Practical aids can help make a person's accommodation suitable for his discharge from hospital. In certain cases, the type of accommodation itself will need to be assessed.

A person may be unable to manage stairs, may now be in a wheelchair, or may have a degree of physical disability which makes managing in the original environment impracticable. Much may depend on the amount of family support that is available. If necessary, alternative arrangements can be made: new housing, a sheltered flat or a local authority home can all be considered.

Follow-up care

It is important for a person to know how his future care is to be arranged. His level of health may need to be observed and his treatment may need to be altered. His general practitioner must be informed abut his discharge and treatment while the person is still in hospital. An out-patient appointment may be given. Unless appropriate follow-up care is organized, ill-health may return.

The above factors should all be considered when a person is discharged from hospital. They should be remembered throughout the admission, so that planning a person's discharge occurs at the beginning of his stay in hospital. Care will be of limited benefit unless people and their problems are related to their environment outside hospital.

Conclusion

In caring for people during their stay in hospital, the nurse must consider them as individuals. They have their own lives outside the hospital. It is all too easy in a busy hospital for a person to become just a patient with a disease in a hospital bed.

The nurse has a vital role in ensuring people are cared for in a way which enhances their independence and personality. She must remember that each person is an individual and not simply a patient.

Further reading

Argyle, M. (1983) *The Psychology of Interpersonal Behaviour,* 4th edition. London: Penguin.

Boore, J. (1978) *Prescription for Recovery* London: Royal College of Nursing.

Bridge, W. & Macleod Clark, J. (1981) *Communication in Nursing Care* London: HM & M.

Hunt, J. & Marks-Maran, D. (1980) *Nursing Care Plans — the Nursing Process at Work* London: HM & M.

Marriner, A. (1983) *The Nursing Process,* 3rd edition. St Louis: C.V.

Roberts, I. (1975) *Discharged from Hospital* London: Royal College of Nursing.

Stockwell, F. (1972) *The Unpopular Patient* London: Royal College of Nursing.

2
Medical Nursing Problems

This chapter deals with the general medical nursing care which may be encountered when caring for patients with a variety of medical disorders. Subsequent chapters will give guidelines to nursing problems specific to the medical condition being considered.

The problem-solving approach allows nurses to care for the patient as an individual. The nurse who takes an accurate admission history will obtain information on which to base an assessment of the patient's problems, identifying the physical, emotional, spiritual and cultural components. She is then in a position to set realistic goals, plan and deliver the required care, and continuously evaluate the effectiveness of this care.

Problems associated with the gastrointestinal tract

Problem A dry, sore or offensive mouth.

Aim To achieve a clean and moist mouth.

Causes

Dehydration	Nil orally
Vomiting	— postoperatively
Infection	— bowel obstruction
— thrush *(Candida albicans)*	Mouth breathing, especially when
— gingivitis	receiving oxygen therapy
— parotitis	Drugs, e.g. atropine
Tooth decay	Vitamin B_{12} deficiency
Ill-fitting dentures	(pernicious anaemia)

Care plan
- Assist the medical staff in treating the cause.
- Increase fluid intake where possible.
- Give mouth care at least hourly initially, and alter the frequency as the mouth improves.

- Offer the patient foods which stimulate the flow of saliva, e.g. pineapple, oranges.
- Prevent cross-infection.
- Explain to the patient how to maintain a clean, moist mouth.

Most patients are able to drink freely, and to clean their own teeth with a toothbrush and toothpaste. When the patient is unable to make proper use of these, or of a mouthwash, mouth care should be given using foam-tipped or cottonwool-tipped mouthsticks, or forceps and swabs. Sodium bicarbonate (5 ml in 300 ml of water) is useful for removing crusts. Soft paraffin can be used to lubricate dry areas. A soft toothbrush may be effective for cleaning a very coated tongue. Dentures, if present, should be removed and cleaned thoroughly.

White patches in the mouth may be due to the yeast-like fungus, *Candida albicans*. In adults it occurs when resistance to infection is low, especially in those receiving antibiotic or steroid therapy. A mouth swab is sent to the laboratory in order to confirm the presence of infection with *Candida albicans* (thrush). Frequent mouth care is given and the patient should have his own feeding utensils to prevent cross-infection. Treatment is with nystatin suspension, amphotericin lozenges or miconazole gel, which are given after meals as they act locally.

Problem Loss of appetite.

Aim To assist the patient to achieve a good nutritional intake.

Causes

Physical or psychological illness
Unpleasant taste in the mouth
Sore mouth, infections
Unappetizing, poorly presented food
No teeth
Gastrointestinal disturbance
— nausea
— vomiting
— dyspepsia
— diarrhoea
— constipation
Pain
Anxiety

Cultural and religious differences making hospital food unacceptable, for example:
— Hinduism
— Sikhism
— Islam
— Orthodox Jewish
Immobilization
— arms
— legs
— lying flat

Care plan

- Assist the medical staff in treating the cause.
- Assist the patient with the care of his mouth at least two-hourly.
- Ensure that the patient is wearing his dentures.
- Offer small attractive meals every two to three hours.
- Discover the patient's likes and dislikes by referring to the nursing history and by further observation and information gathering.
- Relieve pain and anxiety.
- Provide the patient with his appropriate ethnic diet.
- Assist the patient with feeding. This includes:
    correct positioning
    easily accessible tables
    cutting up large pieces of food
    soft diet if the patient has no teeth
    a good choice of food where possible — 'a little of what you fancy does you good'

The patient's nutritional requirements may be altered during the course of his illness. When fever or infection is present, there is an increased metabolic rate. Toxins suppress the appetite and if illness is prolonged and nutritional intake inadequate, malnutrition may occur.

During an acute illness, food should be fluid or semi-fluid at first. Milk, eggs, cooked cereals and custards are useful foods in such cases. The fluid intake should be two to three litres a day unless contraindicated. Later the patient may appreciate a light diet such as creamed chicken, fish, puréed vegetables, or stewed fruit.

Vitamin supplements may be necessary if the illness lasts for some time. If bed rest is prolonged, demineralization of bones may occur because the normal weight-bearing areas are not being used. A good calculation of fluid intake is essential to prevent formation of renal calculi.

Problem Vomiting.

Aim To alleviate vomiting or to promote comfort.

Causes
Infection
— food poisoning
— systemic infection
Dietary indiscretions, e.g. over-indulgence in alcohol
Poisons
Drugs, for example:
— morphine
— cytotoxic drugs
Stress
Disorders of the gastrointestinal tract, for example:
— peptic ulceration
— obstruction
— hiatus hernia
Side-effect of other disorders
— renal failure
— cardiac failure
Radiation
Pregnancy

Care plan
● Assist the medical staff in treating the cause.
● Perform mouth care frequently.
● Measure fluid intake, loss and vomit.
● Give small frequent meals.
● Avoid fats.
● Maintain adequate fluid intake.
● Alleviate stress.
● Control pain.
● Give anti-emetic drugs, for example:
     metoclopramide
     prochlorperazine
     cyclizine

Small, well-presented meals may help the patient to regain his appetite. If these are not tolerated and vomiting is prolonged, the patient may need intravenous fluid and electrolyte replacement.

Problem Constipation.

Aim To achieve a normal bowel action.

Causes

Immobility
Diet deficient in roughage
Dehydration
Pain
Stress, embarrassment
Drugs, for example:
— codeine
— sedatives
— morphine

Mechanical problems in bowel,
e.g. obstruction
Loss of bowel habit through
over-use of aperients
Other medical diseases, e.g.
hypothyroidism

Constipation can cause confusion in the elderly. It causes discomfort in any age group.

Care plan
● Assist the medical staff in treating the cause.
● Increase the mobility of the patient.
● Allow the patient to use the lavatory rather than the bedpan.
● Increase the roughage content of the diet by adding bran, cereals, fruit, vegetables and wholemeal bread.
● Increase fluid intake if possible.
● Give aperients, suppositories or enemas.

Aperients which are commonly used include faecal softeners such as Mil-Par or liquid paraffin, bulk purgatives such as methyl-cellulose or Isogel, or disaccharides such as lactulose. Dorbanex, senna and bisacodyl (Dulcolax) are also used. Glycerine or bisacodyl suppositories are inserted into the rectum and should be retained for about twenty minutes.

The most commonly used enema is sodium phosphate, which is supplied in a disposable sachet. This should be inserted high up at the side of the rectum and retained for about twenty minutes.

Occasionally retention enemas such as arachis oil may be necessary to soften the faeces.

Problem Diarrhoea.

Aim To achieve a normal bowel action.

Causes
Infection
— food poisoning

— loss of normal flora due to antibiotic therapy
— generalized infection
— cholera and dysentery

Disorders of the gastrointestinal tract, for example:
— ulcerative colitis
— malabsorption
— Crohn's disease

Disorders of other organs, for example:
— renal failure
— cardiac failure

Dietary indiscretions
Overuse of aperients
Stress
Constipation with overflow

Care plan

● Assist the medical staff in treating the cause.
● Give milk, milk puddings, yoghurt, etc. in the diet, and avoid unripe fruit and vegetables.
● Increase the fluid intake to replace the loss.
● Prevent excoriation of the anal area by application of a barrier cream or silicone spray.
● Use drugs which slow intestinal motility, for example:
    kaolin and morphine
    codeine phosphate
    loperamide
    Lomotil
    Colofac
● Take care when handling bedpans in case infection is present.
● Provide easy access to the lavatory.

If the diarrhoea is severe, oral dextrose and saline solutions may be used. Fluid and electrolyte replacement by the intravenous route is necessary when dehydration is present. Bed rest will help to reduce the frequency of bowel action. Fluid intake and loss should be measured. The frequency of stools should be recorded in order to assess the effectiveness of the treatment.

If infection is suspected, a specimen of faeces should be sent to the laboratory for culture and sensitivity. Isolation may be necessary to prevent cross-infection.

Problem Faecal incontinence.

Aim To assist the patient to become continent or to achieve comfort and social confidence.

Causes
Loss of consciousness
Loss of control over sphincter
— paralysis
— ageing
Diarrhoea or constipation with overflow
Stress
Apathy

Care plan
- Assist the medical staff in treating the cause.
- Wash and dry skin after episodes of incontinence.
- Apply barrier cream to prevent excoriation.
- Regulate bowel habit by a high roughage diet.
- Establish a routine for the patient by taking him to the lavatory at regular intervals.
- Alleviate stress and embarrassment by providing easy access to the lavatory and easily removable clothing.

Suppositories or enemas can be used to regulate the bowel habit. If these are ineffective, manual evacuation of the rectum may be necessary.

Problems associated with the renal tract

Problem Difficulty in passing urine.

Aim To assist the patient to pass normal amounts of urine painlessly. The normal volume should be ascertained from the nursing history.

Causes

Infection (cystitis)	Drugs
Obstruction	— anaesthesia
— prostatic enlargement	— ephedrine
— calculi	Stress
Haematuria with clots	Dehydration
After pelvic surgery	

Care plan
- Assist the medical staff in treating the cause.

- Increase fluid intake to at least three litres/day (fluid restrictions may be imposed in some disorders of the kidneys, heart and liver).
- Alleviate stress by allowing the patient to use the lavatory or commode, or to stand upright.
- Make urine alkaline by giving sodium or potassium citrate mixture. Alkaline urine is less irritant than acidic urine.

Running taps, hot baths, and drinking gin are all remedies which have also been successful for a patient with retention of urine! If the patient does not respond to the measures outlined above, and retention of urine is present, catheterization will be necessary.

Rarely, a neuromuscular drug such as distigmine bromide is used to cause bladder contraction.

Problem Urinary incontinence.

Aim To assist the patient to become continent or to provide practical help to enable him to gain social confidence.

Causes

Loss of consciousness	Urgency
Loss of control over sphincter	— infection
— elderly	— drugs, e.g. diuretics
— confused	Constipation, especially the
— sedatives	elderly
— paralysis	Psychological
— multiple sclerosis	— enuresis
— spina bifida	Mechanical problems
	— stress incontinence

Care plan
- Refer to the plan for faecal incontinence (page 23).
- Ensure the patient maintains an adequate fluid intake.
- Appliances can be used to increase the muscle tone of the sphincter.
- Male patients can use a condom appliance.
- Female patients can use protective pants.
- Catheterization may be necessary if all other measures fail.

It is important to remember that incontinence can be very disabling, both socially and emotionally.

Table 1. 'At-risk' scoring system for pressure sores. Patients who score a total of 14 or less on this scale are considered to be at risk of developing a pressure sore

	Score			
	1	2	3	4
A. General physical condition	Very bad	Poor	Fair	Good
B. Mental state	Stuporous	Confused	Apathetic	Alert
C. Activity	Bed-fast	Chair-bound	Walks with help	Ambulant
D. Mobility	Immobile	Very limited	Slightly limited	Full
E. Incontinence	Double	Usually urinary	Occasionally	Never

From Norton, D., McLaren, R. and Exton-Smith, A. N. (1962) *An Investigation of Geriatric Nursing Problems in Hospital.* With kind permission of the authors and the publishers, The National Corporation for the Care of Old People, London.

Problems associated with the skin

Problem Susceptibility to pressure sores.

An 'at-risk' scoring system, such as that shown in Table 1, can be used to determine which patients are particularly susceptible to pressure sores.

Aim To prevent the formation of pressure sores.

Causes

In the elderly:
  loss of skin resilience
  immobility
  incontinence
  arteriosclerosis
In the debilitated, wasted patient:
  poor nutrition
infections
anaemia
immobility
In the paralysed patient:
loss of sensation
immobility
incontinence

In the unconscious patient:
  immobility
  incontinence
In the oedematous patient:
  loss of skin resilience
In the obese patient:
  respiration
  immobility

In the patient with a splint
or other appliance:
  friction
  immobility

The parts of the body susceptible to pressure sores are those over bony prominences, especially the sacral area, hips, heels, elbows, knees, ankles, shoulders, spine, and back of head.

The effect of unrelieved pressure will be:
  blistering of the skin
  breaking of the skin
  superficial necrosis and ulcer formation
  gangrene
  sloughing

Care plan
- Change position of the patient at least two-hourly.
- Ensure bed clothes are smooth and free from crumbs.
- Wash and dry skin and apply a barrier cream if incontinence occurs.
- Change soiled sheets.
- Avoid trauma by correct lifting and positioning.
- Supply aids to independence, e.g. monkey pole.
- Use appliances to relieve or redistribute pressure, for example:

water pillows	water bed
sorbo rings	low-loss air bed
foam	cradles
gel pads	sheepskins
ripple mattress	

If a pressure sore does occur it should be treated aseptically. A solution of Eusol or chloramine is useful for cleaning if infection is present. If the sore is deep, it can be packed with ribbon gauze to allow granulation to occur from the base upwards.

Occlusive dressings such as Op-Site or Stomahesive can be applied to superficial sores to promote healing.

Problems associated with body temperature control

Problem Pyrexia — a body temperature above 37.2°C.

Aim If possible to reduce body temperature to within normal limits or to promote comfort.

Causes
Infection
Inflammation
Dehydration
Excessive heat
Cerebral lesions
Necrosis, e.g. myocardial infarction

Care plan
- Assist the medical staff in treating the cause.
- Estimate fluid lost through sweating and increase fluid intake accordingly.
- Perform mouth care at least two-hourly.
- Advise the patient to wear light cotton clothing.
- Advise the patient to rest in bed.
- Give a high-protein, high-calorie diet.
- Fan the patient if his temperature rises above 38°C.
- Change the sheets frequently.
- Give analgesia for headaches and aching joints — aspirin will relieve pain and reduce temperature.
- Record vital signs and maintain an accurate fluid intake and output chart.
- Reduce body temperature by tepid sponging if it rises above 40.5°C.

A *rigor* is an attack of severe shivering associated with a rapid rise in temperature. There are three stages:
1 Uncontrollable shivering as the temperature rises rapidly. The patient feels cold to touch and he has a rapid pulse.
2 Restlessness as the temperature continues to rise. The patient feels very hot and thirsty. His skin is hot and dry. He will often complain of headaches.
3 Profuse sweating followed by a fall in temperature and pulse rate.

The patient should be kept warm during the first stage and should be given hot drinks. During the second stage, blankets should be removed and the patient should be fanned. Cool drinks are helpful. During the third stage, sweat should be wiped from the patient's face, neck and chest to prevent discomfort. Bed clothes should be changed. The patient's temperature should be recorded every 15 minutes throughout the rigor. The patient will appreciate being washed when the rigor is over.

Problem Hypothermia — a body temperature below 35°C.

Aim To restore body temperature to within normal limits.

Causes
Exposure to cold, particularly in the very young and the elderly
— lack of heating
— insufficient clothing
— insufficient food
— immobility
Hypothyroidism (myxoedema), when the body's metabolic rate is reduced
Overdosage of certain drugs, e.g. barbiturates

Care plan
- Assist the medical staff in treating the cause.
- Re-warm the patient slowly in a warm room.
- Cover the patient with an insulating 'space' blanket to preserve heat.
- Give at least three litres of fluid to correct dehydration.
- Assess housing situation and the need for socio-economic support.

Vital signs and the level of consciousness should be monitored. A low-reading rectal thermometer will be necessary to record body temperature. Rapid re-warming should be avoided as vasodilation will cause the blood pressure to drop and heat loss to increase.

Problems associated with maintaining fluid balance

Problem Dehydration.

Aim To rehydrate the patient.

Causes
Insufficient fluid intake
Loss of fluid by
— sweating
— diarrhoea
— vomiting
— excessive urinary output
— rapid respirations
— haemorrhage
— tissue fluid loss, e.g. burns

Care plan
- Assist the medical staff in treating the cause.
- Increase fluid intake by
     oral route
     nasogastric tube
     intravenously
     rectally
- Give frequent mouth care as the mouth will be dry.
- Give pressure area care at least two-hourly.
- Advise the patient to rest in bed.
- Maintain accurate fluid intake and output charts.

Electrolyte imbalance will occur in severe dehydration, and correction will be necessary.

Problem Oedema.

Aim To relieve oedema where possible, and to achieve comfort.

Causes
Cardiac failure
Renal failure
Liver failure
Malignant disease
Malnutrition
Myxoedema
Localized oedema
— injury

— inflammation
— obstruction

Care plan
- Assist the medical staff in treating the cause.
- Restrict salt intake.
- Restrict fluid intake if necessary.
- Weigh the patient daily.
- Maintain accurate fluid intake and output charts.
- Assist the patient to sit upright if pulmonary oedema is present.
- Give pressure area care frequently as the skin will be inelastic.

The specific care of the oedematous patient will be dealt with in the relevant chapters.

Problems associated with pain

The appreciation of the sensation of pain varies from individual to individual. Anxiety, stress, culture or social environment may alter the patient's response to pain.

Aim To relieve pain.

Care plan
- Assist the medical staff in treating the cause.
- Relieve anxiety and stress by explanation.
- Allow the patient to express his feelings about the pain.
- Monitor the level of pain and the effect of analgesia using a pain chart.
- Lift the patient correctly.
- Assist the patient to achieve a comfortable position.
- Apply warmth (or cold) to the affected areas.
- Occupy the patient's attention by conversation, television and games where this is appropriate.
- Give analgesia before pain returns, then adjust the dose down or up to a maintenance level.

Common analgesics are:
   paracetamol or aspirin (weak analgesics)
   codeine or Distalgesic (weak narcotics)

morphine
diamorphine
pethidine
papaveretum
} narcotic analgesia

Vomiting is a common side effect of narcotic analgesia. Anti-emetic drugs may be required.

Achieve comfort by treating other nursing and medical problems such as constipation, dysuria, urinary retention or breathlessness. Alcohol may be given orally in small quantities.

Surgical procedures such as chordotomies (division of an antero-lateral column of the spinal cord) and nerve blocks may be used to relieve pain. Radiotherapy can be used when the cause of pain is malignant disease. Battery-operated stimulators may be used to control sciatic pain.

Problems associated with insomnia

Aim To assist the patient to achieve six hours' sleep in each 24 hours.

Causes
Stress or anxiety
Discomfort
Depression
Noise
Disturbance, e.g. frequent nursing observations
No apparent cause

Care plan
- Assist the medical staff in treating the cause.
- Relieve anxiety by counselling, e.g. listening to problems, explaining procedures.
- Assist the patient to achieve a comfortable position.
- Relieve discomfort and control pain.
- Allow the patient to assume his normal bedtime habits as assessed from the nursing history where this is possible.
- Give alcohol in small quantities, especially to the elderly.
- Give a hot drink or a small meal at bedtime.
- Assist the patient to empty his bladder.
- Give a hypnotic or sedative.

Nitrazepam, diazepam or lorazepam are preferred as hypnotics because they are all safer in overdose than other drugs. Dichloralphenazone (Welldorm) or chloral hydrate are also useful, but can cause gastric irritation. Chlormethiazole (Heminevrin) is useful as a hypnotic and for controlling alcohol withdrawal symptoms.

Barbiturates are rarely used because of the possibility of dependence and the severe effects of overdose.

The elderly may become confused when given hypnotics.

Problems associated with loss of consciousness

Causes

Overdose	Infections
— drugs	— meningitis
— alcohol	— encephalitis
Anaesthesia	— systemic infections
Cerebrovascular accident	Hypoglycaemia
Cerebral tumours	Electrolyte imbalance
Head injury	Respiratory distress
Epilepsy	Renal failure (uraemia)
Liver failure	Endocrine disease

Problem 1 Inability to maintain own airway.

Aim To maintain a clear airway and ensure an adequate oxygen supply to all tissues.

Care plan
● Remove dentures.
● Position the patient so that his tongue does not fall backwards.
● Place the patient in a semi-prone or lateral position.
● Alter the patient's position at least two-hourly to prevent stasis in the lungs.
● Perform pharyngeal or tracheal suction to clear secretions.
● Observe the patient to detect deterioration in his respiratory rate and depth.
● Observe the patient to detect the development of cyanosis.

If there is respiratory embarrassment, a Guedal airway can be inserted. Severe respiratory distress may necessitate insertion of an endotracheal tube, the formation of a tracheostomy or mechanical ventilation.

Problem 2 Susceptibility to pressure sores.

Aim To prevent formation of pressure sores.

Care plan See page 26.

Problem 3 Inability to maintain personal hygiene.

Aim To maintain cleanliness of skin, hair, nails, mouth, and eyes.

Care plan
● Wash and dry skin.
● Keep nails clean and short.
● Comb hair regularly and wash as necessary.
● Perform mouth care at least two-hourly.
● Remove and clean oral airway at least two-hourly.
● Clean eyes with sterile cottonwool balls soaked in warm isotonic saline.
● Prevent risk of injury to eyes due to lack of sensation.
● Shave male patients daily.

Problem 4 Inability to maintain nutritional state.

Aim To provide adequate nutrition and fluids.

Care plan
● Feed the patient by the nasogastric or the intravenous route.
● See also Chapter 10.

Drugs may be given in liquid form via a nasogastric tube or by intravenous injection.

Problem 5 Urinary incontinence or retention.

Aim To prevent occurrence of incontinence and retention.

Care plan
● Express the patient's bladder manually every two hours.

- Use appliances
    condoms
    catheterization
- Reduce risk of urinary tract infections by
    strict aseptic catheterization procedure
    catheter hygiene at least four-hourly
    adequate fluid intake

Problem 6 Constipation or faecal incontinence.

Aim To achieve a regular bowel action.

Care plan
- Give enemas or suppositories every three days.
- Manually evacuate the bowel.
- Add bran to nasogastric feeds.
- Avoid secondary infection via nasogastric feeds.

Problem 7 Immobility.

Aim To prevent stiffening of joints, contractures, muscle wasting, foot-drop and venous thrombosis. To prevent stasis of secretions, which may lead to chest infection, and of urine, which may lead to urinary calculi formation.

Care plan
- Perform passive exercise to all joints each time the patient is turned, i.e. at least two-hourly.
- Assist with chest physiotherapy.
- Maintain a fluid intake of at least two litres every 24 hours.

Observation of vital signs is essential in the unconscious patient. Explanation is always important, as is conversation, as the sense of hearing may be present.

The personal care of the patient should be performed with dignity and without unnecessary exposure. The patient's relatives will need continual support.

Further reading

Billing, H. (1981) *Practical Procedures for Nurses,* 3rd edition. London: Baillière Tindall.

Clarke, M. (1983) *Practical Nursing,* 13th edition. London: Baillière Tindall.

Collins, S. & Parker, E. (1983) *An Introduction to Nursing* London: Macmillan.

Roper, N., Logan, W. & Tierney, A. (1980) *The Elements of Nursing* Edinburgh: Churchill Livingstone.

Storrs, A. (1980) *Geriatric Nursing,* 2nd edition. London: Baillière Tindall.

Wells, T.J. (1980) *Problems in Geriatric Nursing Care* Edinburgh: Churchill Livingstone.

3
Care of the Dying

The period of dying may be accompanied by pain, bodily impairment and mental anguish. It is difficult for a person to visualize his own death, and most people have a greater fear of the *process of dying* than the *fact of death*. The nurse has an important role in allaying these fears and anxieties.

Where possible it is best for people who are dying to be cared for at home. Familiar surroundings and the nearness of those who are aware of the individual's needs and preferences can ease the fear felt. Support can be given by the community nurses or the domiciliary nurses attached to hospices.

Recent years have seen the development of hospices for the terminally ill. These are centres specializing in the care of people who are dying. They provide a model on which nurses within hospitals should base their care.

There is perhaps a danger that, instead of learning from these specialist centres, nurses will leave the proper care of the dying to them, the thinking being that if you have a renal disease you go to a renal unit, and if you are dying you go to a hospice. However, as most deaths take place within a hospital setting, nurses must not abandon their role in these circumstances. Caring for people who are dying is an integral part of nursing. The skills and attitudes developed in the hospice movement can be used to give good care within hospital wards.

The aim of this chapter is to outline some of the ways in which a nurse can help the person who is dying. The areas that will be considered are:

● Psychological care
● Spiritual care
● Family involvement and support
● 'To tell or not to tell'
● The needs of the nursing staff
● Physical care

This is only an introduction to nursing people who are dying. It is important that all nurses develop their skills by further reading, through their education programme, and by practical involvement.

Psychological care

The psychological response to dying involves certain characteristic stages. Dr Elizabeth Kübler-Ross has described five stages of grief a person may experience on learning he has a fatal illness. They are defence mechanisms, and an awareness of these stages will help the nurse to anticipate and alleviate the person's fears.

Denial
People develop the feeling that 'it can't be true'. This enables them to collect themselves and come to terms with the information. Denial is normally a holding pattern and will soon be replaced by partial acceptance.

Nursing intervention Listening is important at this stage. People should be allowed to day-dream about happier things. Denial will fade if they are aware that someone will be available to help them express their feelings when they are ready.

Anger
When denial fades it can be replaced by anger and rage — 'Why me?' This anger may be directed at many different things. Nurses are often the target for this anger and 'can do nothing right'. It is almost as if the person is saying 'I'm not dead yet'.

Nursing intervention This is a difficult period as the anger will be directed towards all sorts of things: the food may be poor, the bed badly made, the nurses may do everything wrong, the doctors don't know what they are talking about, and so on. The nurse must remember why the person is angry. The anger must not be taken personally. It is a generalized feeling of frustration and rage which is displaced onto individual things and people.

It is important to understand what is happening and to give the person time to express his emotion. His anger will then fade. It is all too easy to take this behaviour personally, and to avoid the person, but this may only increase his anger as it leaves no one to attack. The provision of time and attention will allow the person to work through his feelings.

Bargaining
This is a stage where people may try to enter into an agreement with someone or something in an attempt to postpone the inevitable. It is usually a brief period.

Nursing intervention Many of the bargains may be unexpressed. The individual may make them with himself, or with his God. The nurse must ensure that his spiritual needs are being met, and this may be an appropriate time to involve the relevant religious authority or adviser.

Depression
Denial and anger may be replaced by a great sense of loss or sadness. This is perhaps a preparatory grief that the person needs to suffer before his final separation. It may focus on a past or impending loss.

Nursing intervention The nurse must allow time for grieving. Non-verbal communication can be particularly helpful. Sitting with people and holding their hands can mean more than words; so can the expression on one's face. Again, providing time is important. Encouragement, reassurance and telling people not to feel sad is *unhelpful*. They will naturally be sad and one should share that feeling and not deny its validity. These feelings are necessary if the person is to reach the final stage of acceptance.

Acceptance
A person who has had the time and help to work through these stages will reach a point when he is neither depressed nor angry. Having expressed his rage and sense of loss, he reaches a stage of quiet acceptance. This is not a stage of giving up, but a period almost void of feelings.

Nursing intervention This stage is often characterized by tiredness, weakness and long periods of sleep. Again, non-verbal communication is vital. Sitting in silence with the person to show him that you are still there and that you care is important. Touching him, holding his hands or straightening his pillows will help provide comfort.

These stages do not always occur in sequence and may overlap each other. An awareness of these defence mechanisms should guide the nurse's approach and care.

Throughout these stages it is important that the nurse allows the person the time and the opportunity to express his feelings. It is all too easy for nursing to be reduced to the completion of physical tasks, while the nurse, with her own anxieties, avoids the psychological care of the individual.

If possible, nursing people in side rooms should be avoided. This arrangement can make it too easy for nurses to go in, complete their tasks and leave, avoiding the person. People are often nursed in side rooms to allay the anxieties of the nursing staff, rather than for their own benefit. Care and involvement should be *increased* and not withdrawn because someone is terminally ill.

Spiritual care

People's spiritual needs may be of the greatest importance to them during this period. A nurse should know from the nursing history, and from her relationship with her patient, whether he has religious beliefs.

In our multi-cultural society, religious beliefs vary considerably. If a nurse is unable to meet and help with any individual's beliefs, it is important that she ensures they are met by others. Members of the family may be able to provide spiritual support. More particularly, the relevant religious authority or adviser should be involved. In addition to helping the person and their family directly, he will provide guidance for the nurses so as to ensure that their nursing intervention conforms to the person's religious beliefs.

Family involvement and support

The nurse cannot give valid help and support to the person who is dying unless she also considers his family. Their feelings will include hopelessness, anger, isolation and sadness. They may well experience some or all of the psychological stages mentioned previously. Unless the family's feelings are expressed and understood, the individual will be nursed in a vacuum. The care of him as a whole person will suffer accordingly.

Psychological support can be given by involving the family in physical care. Carrying out certain procedures and tasks can ease feelings of helplessness. Washing, positioning, giving medication and making beds, for example, can be done by a nurse and a member of the family together. They should be directly involved in caring. It must always be remembered that the dying person is their spouse, child or other close relative.

The spouse is often the first person to be informed of the severity of the illness and to be told that death may occur. He or she is often then left, without support, to tell the rest of the family. The nurse can help by informing and involving all the family.

The nurse must provide the time to listen to family anxieties and emotions, and must be able to explain what is happening. She should also act as a bridge between the person who is dying and his family, helping them to communicate with each other. The person who is dying may be able to help his family accept his situation by discussing his feelings with them.

Difficulties with visiting, staying at the hospital, leaving children at home, finances or legal concerns can all cause anxiety at such a time. The involvement of social workers or other members of the family may help to ease these worries.

The nurse should also be aware of what support there will be for the immediate family after the death. Bereavement counselling and support from social workers can help ease the feelings that will occur. The nurse must remember that the family's feelings will not end with the person's death.

The degree of family involvement and support will obviously vary on each occasion. The principle remains, however, that, without their involvement, the care of the patient will suffer.

'To tell or not to tell'

Should people who are dying be told? This is a question often raised in nursing. Kübler-Ross says that the question should not be 'Should we tell them what is wrong?', but rather, 'How can we share this information with the person?' This approach is admirable. It establishes a different relationship to that which commonly exists. One can listen to the person for cues about his willingness to know more. It is an empathetic way of relating, developing a relationship based on confidence and trust.

It is important that this sharing of knowledge is accompanied by an assurance that the person will not be abandoned. He must be reassured that everything possible will still be done to maintain his dignity and relieve specific problems.

Both Elizabeth Kübler-Ross and Cicely Saunders (see Further Reading list) would argue that the majority of people are aware of their impending death, whether they have been told or not. People pick up this knowledge from the behaviour of their family, the nurses and the doctors. They can sense a change in approach and any tendency to avoid them and their problems.

Given these facts, the nurse should constantly be aware of how much information the person wishes to share, and should always be sensitive to the timing of communication. The concept of sharing knowledge means that some people will know explicitly and others implicitly what is wrong. This is not telling lies but sharing knowledge according to the wishes of the person who is dying.

The needs of the nursing staff

Caring for the dying creates anxiety and stress among nurses. They may have had little or no experience of death; their own feelings may be unexplored and their means of supporting one another are often poor. As a result, the care they provide for those who are dying may be inadequate.

Within the setting of a ward, nursing staff can share feelings in a supportive way. Discussing what one feels — be it anger, impotence, helplessness, sadness, or a combination of any of these — is necessary when caring for a person who is dying. This must be done openly. Many feelings can be difficult to express as people are worried about what others will think — 'How can I say I dislike or get fed up with someone who is dying?' These feelings may be experienced by others, and only by discussing them together and sharing them can nurses give each other help and support. This can be done either on a one-to-one basis or at meetings of ward staff.

Nurses must be aware of the stress they will experience when nursing people who are dying, and of the emotional demands with which they will have to cope. Unless nurses can discuss and explore their feelings, the care they give will suffer.

Physical care

The person who is dying may have a variety of physical problems caused by his disease (or diseases). Common problems include:

pain	lethargy and weakness
anorexia	pressure sores
nausea and vomiting	insomnia
dry mouth	constipation
hiccup	diarrhoea
dyspnoea	urinary frequency
cough	urinary incontinence

The nursing intervention for these problems is outlined in Chapter 2.

The role of the nurse is vital in the context of these problems, and involves constant assessment and observation. The dying person's general condition means that specific problems can arise very suddenly. The nurse must continually assess the person to anticipate problems. Any problems that cannot be anticipated must be alleviated quickly. This is important, not only to relieve the particular discomfort, but to reassure the person that he has not been abandoned. It emphasizes the philosophy that, although nothing can be done to change the final outcome, this does not mean that there is nothing to be done at all.

If nursing and medical intervention can minimize a person's physical suffering, he will then be free to concentrate on other matters.

Pain in people who are dying

Pain in those who are terminally ill serves no useful purpose. The aim of care should be to ensure that no pain is experienced.

Pain is a wholly subjective symptom. It is impossible to devise a system whereby the nurse can determine the degree of pain felt, yet is is necessary to assess the pain in order to ensure it is controlled. The only reliable method is to ask the person.

A pain observation chart has been designed to help make the

assessment of pain more systematic. The person is asked about his pain at regular intervals, and the nurse records the location and severity of the pain on the chart. This enables the effectiveness of analgesia to be closely monitored. If analgesia is being given regularly, it is necessary to make an observation with each dose, and another half-way between each dose. This is because analgesia must be organized so as to stop pain being experienced before the next dose is given. The memory or fear of pain returning must be prevented as well as the pain itself.

To use the chart, ask the person to mark *all* his pains on the body diagram (Figure 5). It is important to note that pain is often felt in more than one area. Label each site of pain with a letter (A, B, C, etc.). Once this initial assessment has been made, systematic recordings can be carried out on subsequent occasions. At each observation time:

1 Ask the person to assess the pain at each separate site since the last observation. Using the scale with the body diagram (Figure 5) enter the number or letter in the appropriate column of the pain chart (Figure 6).

2 Record the overall pain since the last observation. Use the same scale and enter the level of pain in the column marked 'overall'.

3 Record what nursing measures have been taken to relieve pain.

4 Record the analgesia given.

5 Note any comment on pain from the person or the nursing staff.

This is a means of communication to be used with the person and not on him. It may be helpful if he fills in the chart himself.

Many terminally ill people suffer from cancer and may experience very severe pain. As a result they may be prescribed powerful analgesics such as diamorphine and morphine.

Analgesia is given orally where possible. If vomiting, weakness or dysphagia makes this difficult, drugs can be given rectally or by injection. Where injections are required, they no longer need to be given every three or four hours, but can be given by a syringe pump. A 24-hour dose of an analgesic drug is drawn into a syringe, to which a cannula with a butterfly needle is attached. This syringe is fitted into a pump, which is set to compress the syringe barrel at a steady rate and empty the syringe over 24 hours. The butterfly needle is inserted subcutaneously, and the pump may be fitted into

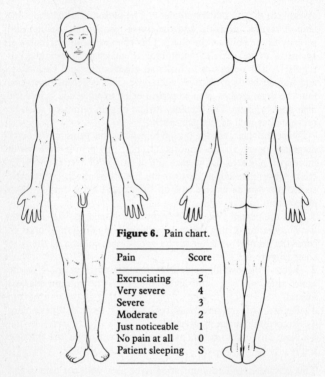

Figure 6. Pain chart.

Pain	Score
Excruciating	5
Very severe	4
Severe	3
Moderate	2
Just noticeable	1
No pain at all	0
Patient sleeping	S

Figure 5. Body diagram and scoring system for assessing pain.

a holster or pouch which fits under the arm or around the waist (Figure 7). Excellent pain control can be achieved by this method. The analgesic, usually diamorphine, is combined with an anti-emetic such as prochlorperazine. The syringe is recharged each day and the needle site is altered after 48 hours.

In addition to the wide choice of analgesic drugs available, the nurse must not neglect the range of nursing measures which help to alleviate pain (see page 30).

The importance of pain control cannot be overstated. Pain can be the most important problem for the person who is dying, clouding everything else.

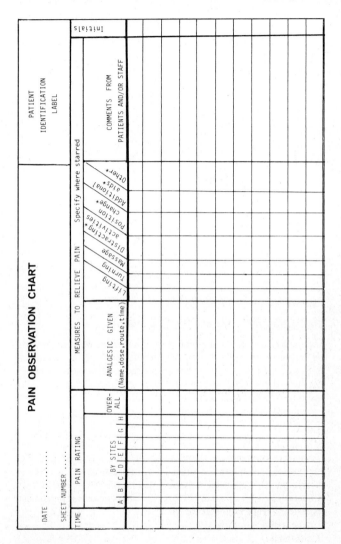

Figure 6. Pain chart.

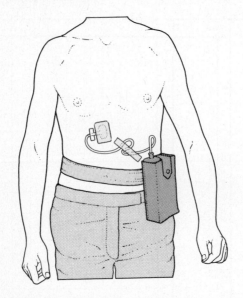

Figure 7. Continuous analgesia.

Radiotherapy in people who are dying

During the last period of a person's life, palliative radiotherapy can be given to relieve distressing problems. If radiotherapy is indicated it should be performed with the lowest possible dose in the fewest possible treatments. The problems that palliative radiotherapy can help with are:

    pain, particularly from bone metatases

    bleeding — haemoptysis, haematuria or vaginal bleeding

    cough and dyspnoea, particularly from bronchial carcinoma

This form of treatment should only be undertaken if an easier method of controlling the problem is impracticable. The area to which radiotherapy is to be applied will be marked — usually with a mauve cross on the skin (Figure 8). The problems a person can experience from radiotherapy are:

    nausea and vomiting

    diarrhoea

    skin damage

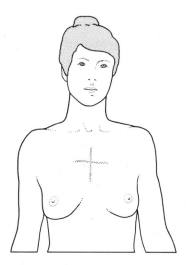

Figure 8. Radiotherapy marking.

Nursing intervention

Nausea and vomiting:

- Give anti-emetics half-an-hour before treatment is due.
- Give anti-emetics before meals. In some cases it may be necessary to give these intramuscularly.
- Ensure that there is a receiver within easy reach.
- Give mouthwashes after vomiting has occurred.

Diarrhoea:

- Give drugs to control diarrhoea, e.g. codeine phosphate or kaolin.
- Ensure easy access to the lavatory or to a commode.

Skin damage:

- Do not wash area marked for radiotherapy. The skin is fragile at this point and rubbing can cause severe skin damage. For the same reason, powders and creams are not applied. These precautions should continue for seven to ten days after completion of radiotherapy.

Conclusion

Wherever possible, people should be nursed at home and cared for by their families. The environment is familiar and the person is appreciated as an individual. His anxieties and fears will be reduced. However, only a small number of dying people can be cared for in this way. Most deaths take place within a hospital, and therefore nurses have a responsibility to become skilled at caring for people who are dying.

It must *never* be assumed that terminal care consists merely of routines performed when there is nothing more to be done. It should not be seen as the end product of failed medical treatment. If this is allowed to happen, the person will feel abandoned and his deepest needs will be ignored. Rather, nurses should try to provide positive help during this period of his life.

Caring for people who will recover alongside those who will not is sometimes regarded as impossible. Care, however, is individual. Nurses must learn to adapt their care to the needs of each person and avoid employing a generalized, blanket approach. In order to do this they must understand the specific physical and psychological needs of the individual who is dying. This understanding must involve the members of his family, each of which will also have their own particular needs.

Nurses have a positive role in allaying anxiety and fears about the process of dying. They have the opportunity to help the person live this part of his life without physical distress and with dignity.

Further reading

Bond, M. (1979) *Pain* Edinburgh: Churchill Livingstone.
Hayward, J.C. (1975) *Information — A Prescription Against Pain* London: Royal College of Nursing.
Hinton, J. (1971) *Dying* London: Penguin.
Kübler-Ross, E. (1973) *On Death and Dying* London: Tavistock.
Parkes, C.M. (1972) *Bereavement — Studies of Grief in Adult Life* London: Tavistock.
Saunders, C. (1978) *The Management of Terminal Disease* London: Edward Arnold.
Speck, P. (1978) *Loss and Grief in Medicine* London: Baillière Tindall.
Tschudin, V. (1982) *Counselling Skills for Nurses* London: Baillière Tindall.

4
Infectious Diseases Nursing

Infection

Infection occurs when a sufficient number of pathogenic micro-organisms reach a susceptible site, multiply and cause an adverse reaction in the host. Pathogenic micro-organisms include bacteria, viruses or fungi.

Infection may be endogenous or exogenous. Endogenous infection originates from organisms normally present in or on the patient. Exogenous infection originates from organisms outside of the patient. The human body has the ability to protect itself from infection; this is known as resistance.

Bacteria are composed of one cell only. Rates of reproduction vary from a few minutes to a few days. Some bacteria are dependent on oxygen (aerobic), while others can thrive without oxygen (anaerobic). Bacteria release toxins into the bloodstream. These toxins may produce local tissue damage or widespread symptoms.

Viruses are much smaller than bacteria and can only reproduce inside a living cell which the virus has invaded. They may spread via the lymphatics and the bloodstream and cause symptoms of infection.

Fungi most commonly cause local infection of the mucous membranes, skin or hair. Rarely generalized infection may occur.

Spread of infection
Sources of infection include:
1 Infected people who have clinical signs of infection. These may include patients, visitors or staff.
2 Carriers who show no signs of infection.
3 Those who are incubating an infection.
4 A reservoir of infection, which occurs in places where organisms can survive and multiply. In a hospital these reservoirs may include sinks, drains, stagnant fluid (e.g. flower vases), dust, contaminated lotions, or organic matter.

Organisms may be spread via:
  direct contact
  food
  blood
  insects
  air
  soil

Some people are more susceptible to infection than others. These include the very young or very old, those with malignant or chronic disease, and those receiving radiotherapy. Other people may have a defective immune system because of disease or drugs such as immunosuppressives or steroids. Patients who have undergone surgery or who have suffered trauma in any way are also susceptible to infection.

Hospital-acquired infection

The hospital environment encourages infection to occur. There is a large number of people together, many of whom are already infected or who are susceptible to infection. There are also many reservoirs of infection in a hospital. More and more of the pathogenic micro-organisms found in hospital are becoming resistant to antibiotics. The most commonly seen infections in a hospital are:
  wound infections
  urinary tract infections
  chest infections

Wound infections can be transmitted on the hands of doctors, nurses or patients, by spread from nose or throat, or by the use of contaminated equipment. Early detection of wound infection is necessary to prevent it spreading to other patients.

Urinary tract infections are usually caused by the patient's own intestinal bacteria. Patients who are confined to bed are more susceptible because of urinary stasis. Catheterization or any instrumentation of the bladder increases the risk of infection. The most commonly responsible are *Escherichia coli, Proteus, Streptococcus faecalis, Klebsiella* and *Pseudomonas*.

Chest infections often occur in patients who have difficulty in breathing because of pain, illness or immobility. Retention of secretions predisposes to infection. The most common organisms involved are *Pneumococcus, Staphylococcus aureus* and *Klebsiella pneumoniae.*

Treatment of infection

Antimicrobial drugs are used to combat infections caused by bacteria, viruses and fungi. These drugs either destroy the micro-organism or prevent its reproduction. Antimicrobial drugs which can destroy many different organisms are said to have a *broad spectrum* of action.

Resistance to certain antimicrobial drugs can develop and a valuable drug may thus become useless. In order to prevent resistance occurring, many hospitals restrict the number of antimicrobial drugs in general use.

Antibiotics are bactericidal drugs. The most common groups of antibiotics are:

1 Penicillins, e.g. flucloxacillin, amoxycillin, penicillin V, benzylpenicillin, and carbenicillin. These drugs are mostly used in the treatment of sensitive staphylococcal infections, gonorrhea and syphilis. Side-effects include rash, infection with *Candida,* diarrhoea, fever, or occasionally anaphylactic shock.

2 Cephalosporins, e.g. cephalexin. These drugs are used in the treatment of penicillin-resistant staphylococcal and streptococcal infections. They are also used for urinary tract infections.

3 Tetracyclines are broad-spectrum antibiotics, but many organisms are now becoming resistant to them.

4 Aminoglycosides, e.g. gentamicin, tobramycin. These drugs are used in serious, sensitive infections. Vestibular disturbances or renal failure may occur if the blood level of the drug is too high.

Other common antibiotics include fucidic acid, chloramphenicol, erythromycin, metronidazole and trimethoprin.

Sulphonamides are bacteriostatic drugs effective against streptococcal, meningococcal, pneumococcal and *E. coli* infections. They are especially used in the treatment of urinary tract infections. Side-effects include fever and allergy. Combinations of sulphonamides and trimethoprin are particularly effective.

Antituberculosis drugs include isoniazid, rifampicin, and ethambutol.

Antifungal drugs include nystatin (which is used in the treatment of *Candida* infections), amphotericin B and griseofulvin.

Antiviral drugs include amandatin and vidarakine.

Immunity

Some individuals, although exposed to infection, do not develop the disease because they already possess effective antibodies. Immunity may be active or passive.

Active immunity may be acquired naturally by having the infection, or artificially by being vaccinated with a harmless form of the antigen.

Passive immunity is short-lived. It may be acquired naturally by the fetus from its mother or artificially by injection of antibodies (gamma globulin).

Vaccination is routinely given to prevent the following infectious diseases:

diphtheria
tetanus
pertussis (whooping cough)
polio
measles
tuberculosis
rubella (German measles)

Infectious diseases

Most individuals who develop the minor communicable diseases do not require admission to hospital. However, those with more serious infections do require nursing, sometimes within an infectious diseases unit. The incidence of serious infections has fallen since the development of antibiotics and the improvement of social conditions, although there are now more 'imported' diseases as a result of increased travel abroad.

Medical and nursing problems

Fever	Skin irritation
Rigors	Rash
Sweating	Diarrhoea
Febrile convulsions	Exhaustion
Dehydration	Confusion
Anorexia	Risk of spread of the infection
Weight loss	

Medical investigation and treatment
• Soluble aspirin (300–600 mg orally, or in suppository form) is

given to reduce pyrexia and to relieve headache and joint pains.
- Diazepam (5–10 mg in adults) may be given to treat persistent rigors or febrile convulsions.
- Intravenous fluids and electrolytes may be neccessary to correct severe dehydration and electrolyte imbalance.
- Chlorpheniramine (4 mg orally) can be given to relieve skin irritation.
- Nystatin suspension or amphotericin lozenges are given to treat oral candidiasis.
- Specimens of stool and urine, and swabs from the ear, nose, throat and skin lesions will be required for microscopy, culture and sensitivity.
- Staff are vaccinated against any serious infectious disease before nursing the patient.
- The Medical Officer of Environmental Health should be informed of a notifiable disease.

Nursing intervention
- The temperature can be reduced by fanning or by tepid sponging. The temperature is recorded at least every two to four hours and more frequently during tepid sponging.
- Dehydration, resulting from sweating, vomiting, diarrhoea and increased metabolism, is corrected. An adult is encouraged to drink two-and-a-half to three litres of fluid in 24 hours. An accurate fluid intake and output chart is kept.
- A well-balanced diet is important. High-calorie drinks are encouraged. Milk shakes, soups and milk puddings are often appreciated and are high in protein and calories.
- Attention to hygiene is essential. A daily bed bath is given and sponging is performed as required, throughout the day. Sheets are changed as often as necessary.
- Mouth care is given two-hourly, and the patient may appreciate ice or boiled sweets to suck. The nurse looks for signs of oral *Candida* infection presenting as white spots in the mouth.
- The patient's position is changed at least two-hourly to prevent skin damage. Calamine lotion may be applied to an irritating skin rash.
- The frequency, colour, consistency and quantity of the patient's bowel action is recorded if there is diarrhoea. Careful washing and drying of the skin is essential after episodes of

incontinence, and a barrier cream such as zinc and castor oil may be applied to prevent excoriation of the skin.

- Rest is important for a patient who has an infectious disease and disturbance should be minimized. Sedation may be necessary, especially if confusion is present.

- The danger of spread of infection varies according to the micro-organisms involved. Some patients may need to be nursed in an infectious diseases unit.

- When a patient is nursed in a general ward he should have his own room with washbasin and toilet facilities. All persons entering the room should wear plastic aprons or disposable gowns. Masks are rarely necessary unless the disease is spread by droplets.

- Gloves are only required for direct contact with infected tissues. However, handwashing is essential after any contact with the patient.

- Separate bedpans and urinals are necessary. The patient should use disposable crockery and cutlery.

- Cleaning of the room takes place in the usual way but with separate utensils. Linen is placed in special colour-coded bags.

- The room is cleaned thoroughly with hot water and detergent after the patient has vacated it.

Notifiable diseases

The following diseases should be reported by the attending doctor to the appropriate Medical Officer of Environmental Health:

acute encephalitis	ophthalmia neonatorum
acute meningitis	paratyphoid fever
acute poliomyelitis	plague
anthrax	rabies
cholera	relapsing fever
diphtheria	scarlet fever
dysentery	smallpox
food poisoning	tetanus
infective jaundice	tuberculosis
lassa fever	typhoid fever
leprosy	typhus fever
leptospirosis	viral haemorrhagic fever
malaria	whooping cough
Marburg disease	yellow fever
measles	

Sexually transmitted diseases

The most common sexually transmitted diseases in the United Kingdom are gonorrhoea and non-specific urethritis. The incidence of genital herpes simplex is increasing, but the incidence of syphilis is static.

Gonorrhoea
The causative organism is *Neisseria gonorrhoeae* (gonococcus) and this is most often transmitted from one person to another during sexual intercourse.

Since the introduction of the contraceptive pill, there has been a rise in the incidence of gonorrhoea. This increase may be due to the fact that younger women are now more likely to have several sexual partners and more frequent coitus. In addition, the contraceptive sheath, which offers some protection against sexually transmitted diseases, is being used less and less.

The incubation period of gonorrhoea is about three to ten days. In the male, a white or yellow urethral discharge and dysuria develop. In the female these symptoms may be trivial, but ascending infection may cause acute salpingitis. Treatment is with penicillin, although the gonococcus is becoming increasingly resistant to this drug, necessitating the use of broad-spectrum antibiotics.

Non-specific urethritis
The incidence of non-specific urethritis (NSU) has increased over the last few years. Many cases are due to infection with mycoplasma or chlamydia, but in many others no organism can be found. Treatment is with a broad-spectrum antibiotic.

Herpes simplex virus
Approximately 10 000 new cases of genital herpes simplex virus (HSV) occur each year. The severity of symptoms varies. Painful vesicles develop in the genital region and heal about one to four weeks later. Vaginal discharge and dysuria may also occur. The symptoms recur at intervals of anything from a month to a few years.

There is no cure for this unpleasant disease and the patient will need much psychological support. The affected areas should be kept clean and dry. In female patients, soaking in a bath is helpful, drying well afterwards. Simple analgesics may be required. Strict

handwashing is essential. This infection may be transmitted to the
unborn child, causing mental handicap.

Syphilis

Syphilis is caused by the organism *Treponema pallidum*. The
incubation period is ten days to ten weeks. A primary lesion
(chancre) develops at the site of infection, usually on the genitals.
This lesion ulcerates and then tends to heal. In the secondary
stage, rashes, condylomata, 'snail-track' ulcers in the mouth, and
enlarged lymph nodes occur. In the tertiary stage (2–30 years
later), lesions can appear anywhere, e.g. heart, central nervous
system, liver, tongue or bone.

Congenital syphilis occurs when the infection is transmitted
from the mother to the fetus.

Treatment of syphilis is with procaine penicillin.

Septicaemia

Septicaemia is a serious condition in which pathogenic micro-
organisms multiply in the bloodstream. The most common
organisms are *Staphylococcus aureus, Streptococcus pyogenes,
Escherichia coli, Pseudomonas, Klebsiella* and the anaerobic
Bacteriodes.

Septicaemia may originate from infection in the abdomen, ear,
nose, throat or lungs. The patient may be already debilitated by
surgery, immunosuppression or other severe infections.

Fever and rigors occur. The patient may become shocked with a
low blood pressure, confusion and diminished urine output. The
skin is often pink. Pulmonary oedema, acidosis and disturbances
in clotting may occur.

Blood cultures are obtained in order to determine the causative
organism and antibiotics are then given intravenously. Intravenous
fluid and plasma may be require to correct shock.

Gastroenteritis

Gastroenteritis is a common infection caused by *Escherichia,
Shigella sonnei, Campylobacter, Salmonella,* and the rotavirus. It
can be transmitted by faecal–oral spread. Food infected by
Salmonella and *Campylobacter* also causes gastroenteritis.

The patient develops a fever and diarrhoea. Dehydration may

result, particularly in babies. The stool is cultured to determine the causative organism.

Gastroenteritis usually resolves spontaneously within a few days. Antibiotic therapy is rarely needed. Rehydration is necessary; an infant should be given a dilute solution of electrolytes and glucose.

In order to prevent gastroenteritis, food should be thoroughly cooked. Hands and working surfaces should be washed with hot water and soap, and dried thoroughly. Cooked foods which have been left and reheated are particularly dangerous.

Malaria

Human malaria results from infection by *Plasmodium falciparum*, *Plasmodium vivax*, *Plasmodium ovale*, or *Plasmodium malariae*. Infection is acquired as a result of a bite from an anopheline mosquito which has itself become infected with the malarial parasite. In the human, the parasites multiply in the liver for six to eleven days until they are released into the blood, producing a fever. A rigor occurs, followed by a hot stage, then a sweating stage. Vomiting and headache often occur. Delirium may accompany the hot stage. In vivax malaria, the fever occurs on alternative days.

Falciparum malaria is a more severe form in which haemolytic anaemia develops and in which cerebral complications may occur.

Malaria is treated with oral chloroquine. Rest is important and the patient should drink two-and-a-half to three-and-a-half litres of fluid in 24 hours. Aspirin or paracetamol is given to relieve headache. Occasionally intravenous fluid replacement is indicated.

Attacks of malaria can be prevented by taking proguanil or pyrimethamine on entering a region where malaria is found. The drugs should be continued regularly until four weeks after leaving the region.

Mosquitoes can be controlled by spraying houses with DDT. Mosquito nets or wire-screened houses are essential in malarial regions.

Conclusion

There has been a decline in the incidence of communicable disease in the UK due to immunization and health education. It is

Table 2. Infectious diseases

Disease	Method of spread	Incubation period (days)	Infectious period	Symptoms and signs	Complications	Treatment
Mumps	Droplet Direct contact or infected food	14–28	Three days before illness until after facial swelling has subsided	Tender swelling of salivary glands Headache Difficulty chewing Fever	Orchitis Oophoritis Pancreatitis Myocarditis	
Chickenpox	Direct contact Droplet	12–24	Six days before illness until all skin lesions are dry	Rash mainly on trunk Groups of spots together developing into vesicles and pustules Fever	Bacterial infection of skin Pneumonia	
Whooping cough	Direct contact Droplet	7–15	Three days before until ten days after cough develops	Catarrh Cough Vomiting Fever Paroxysms of coughing followed by inspiratory 'whoop'	Bronchitis Rupture of blood vessels in eyes, skin or brain Aspiration pneumonia	

Disease	Spread	Incubation	Isolation	Symptoms	Complications	Treatment
Infectious mononucleosis (glandular fever)	Saliva	5–10	Only mildy infectious	Fine rash Fever Sore throat Anorexia Headache	Illness can persist for many weeks or months	
Scarlet fever	Droplet	2–4	Until *Strep. pyogenes* has been cleared from throat	Erythema of face then body Fever Sore throat Vomiting Furred tongue	Peritonsillar abscess Glomerulonephritis Rheumatic fever	Oral penicillin given
Diphtheria	Droplet	2–5	Until throat swab is negative	Headache Sore throat Grey membrane across pharynx Tachycardia Low blood pressure Mild fever Visual disturbances Dysphagia	Respiratory obstruction Involvement of central nervous system and myocardium Pneumonia	Immediate treatment with antitoxin

Table 2 continued

Disease	Method of spread	Incubation period (days)	Infectious period	Symptoms and signs	Complications	Treatment
Smallpox	Droplet Direct contact	12	Until last scab has been shed	Fever Headache Sore throat Ulcers in mouth and throat Rash on face, scalp and limbs Vesicles and pustules Pneumonia	Heart failure Bronchopneumonia Corneal ulcers	Isolation in infectious diseases unit necessary
Typhoid	Contaminated food	7–21	Until six consecutive stool and urine specimens are negative	Anorexia Headache Diarrhoea Vomiting Fever Enlarged spleen Rose pink spots (scattered)	Carrier state in 5% Haemorrhage Perforation of intestine	Isolation in infectious diseases unit necessary Treated with chloramphenicol or ampicillin
Bacillary dysentery	Contaminated food	3–7	Until stool specimens negative	Abdominal pain Diarrhoea Fever	Dehydration	

important to ensure that travellers are vaccinated against any diseases endemic in the region they are visiting. Immigrants should be screened for infectious diseases on arrival in the country. Strict control is enforced on imported food and live animals.

Diseases such as poliomyelitis, diphtheria, tetanus and smallpox are much less common following the widespread use of prophylactic immunization. Malaria has been greatly reduced in many areas, although many more cases are now seen in the UK as a result of travel abroad.

Further reading

Nursing 2 (1982) *Body Defences* Volume 6 (October).
Nursing 2 (1982) *Infection* Volumes 7 and 8 (November and December).
Parker, J. & Stucke, U. (1978) *Microbiology for Nurses*, 5th edition. London: Baillière Tindall.
Parry, W.H. (1979) *Communicable Diseases*, 3rd edition. London: Hodder & Stoughton.
Schofields, C.B.O. (1979) *Sexually Transmitted Diseases* 3rd edition. Edinburgh: Churchill Livingstone.

5
Cardiovascular Nursing

The cardiovascular system consists of the heart and blood vessels. Figure 9 shows the chambers of the heart and the great vessels that enter and leave the heart.

There are three layers of the heart:
  pericardium — outer sac of two coats
  myocardium — muscle tissue
  endocardium — lining

The coronary arteries, which supply the myocardium with blood, are shown in Figure 10.

Contraction of the atria and ventricles is caused by electrical impulses passing along the conducting pathways of the heart.

Investigations

Electrocardiogram
An electrocardiogram (ECG) is the tracing obtained by recording the electrical impulses conducted in the heart muscle. Figure 11 shows a normal ECG.

Echocardiogram
An echocardiogram is a recording of sound waves reflected from surfaces outside and inside the heart. Valve disease can be diagnosed using this technique. The size of the ventricles can also be assessed.

Cardiac catheterization
This procedure involves the passage of a thin, hollow, flexible tube (catheter) into the right or left side of the heart. The catheter is inserted into a vein or artery of the arm of leg. The catheter is

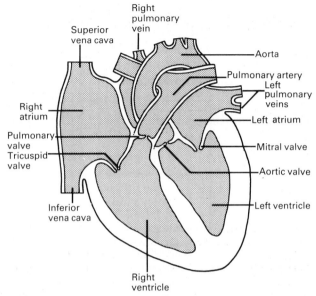

Figure 9. The heart.

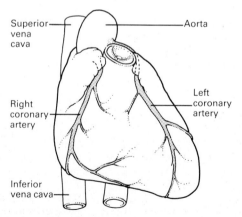

Figure 10. The coronary arteries.

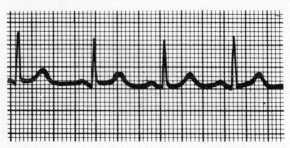

Figure 11. Normal ECG.

radio-opaque and so its insertion can be monitored using X-rays. This technique is used in order to measure the pressures in the vessels and chambers of the heart. Blood samples can be taken for blood gas estimations.

A radio-opaque dye can be injected via the catheter to outline the vessels. This procedure is called angiography.

There are risks associated with cardiac catheterization and careful explanation and consent are necessary. A mild sedative is sometimes given prior to the procedure, which is performed under a local anaesthetic. The patient should have nothing to eat or drink for six hours before the investigation.

The risks of cardiac catheterization are:
   haemorrhage from the site
   arrhythmias
   infection

The insertion site should be observed every 15 minutes for the first few hours. The patient should stay in bed. Direct pressure should be applied if bleeding occurs. The pulse and blood pressure should be recorded every 15 minutes for two hours and then every 30 minutes for four hours. Irregularity of the pulse may indicate arrhythmias. The doctor should be informed of this and of any episodes of chest pain. The temperature should be recorded every four hours. Pyrexia may indicate infection.

Arrhythmias

The normal heart beat is regular. Disturbances in heart rhythm are called arrhythmias. Some of the common arrhythmias are shown below.

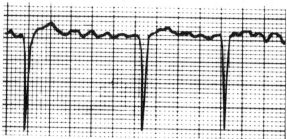

Figure 12. Atrial fibrillation.

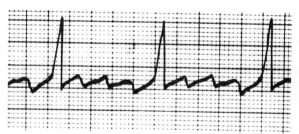

Figure 13. Atrial flutter.

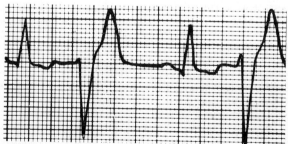

Figure 14. Ventricular ectopics.

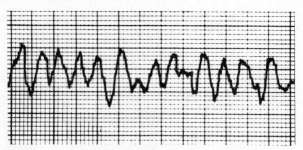

Figure 15. Ventricular fibrillation.

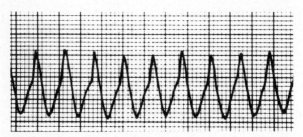

Figure 16. Ventricular tachycardia.

Congenital heart disease

Various forms of abnormality can occur during the development of the heart. Some are mild and can go unnoticed. Some are so severe that the child dies soon after birth. The main types of congenital heart disease are:

Patent ductus arteriosus (Figure 17)
Pulmonary valve stenosis (Figure 18)
Fallot's tetralogy (Figure 19)
— ventricular septal defect
— dextro position of aorta
— pulmonary valve stenosis
— thickened wall of right ventricle
Atrial septal defect (Figure 20)

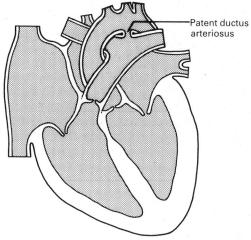

Figure 17. Patent ductus arteriosus.

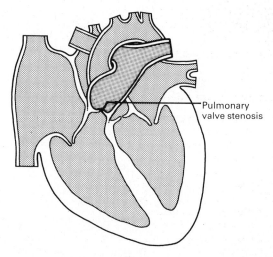

Figure 18. Pulmonary valve stenosis.

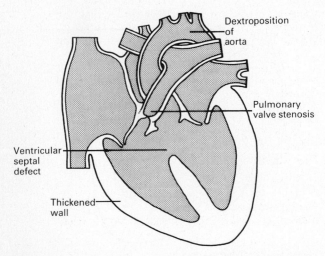

Figure 19. Fallot's tetralogy.

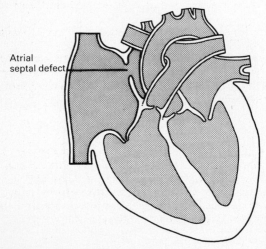

Figure 20. Atrial septal defect.

Causes
Maternal infection in early pregnancy, e.g. rubella
Genetic

Medical and nursing problems
Cyanosis
— if blood is shunted from the right to left side of the heart
Dyspnoea
Clubbing of fingers
Failure to thrive
Heart murmurs
— often noticed at a 'medical'

Medical treatment
Most congenital abnormalities are surgically corrected.

Chronic valvular heart disease

This condition occurs mainly as a result of inflammation of the valve cusps, leading to distortion, fibrosis and calcification of the valve.

Chronic valvular disease often occurs as a result of rheumatic fever (see Chapter 12, page 208).

Stenosis is a narrowing of the valve. *Incompetence* is inadequate closure of the valve. *Regurgitation* is backflow of blood as a result of incompetence. Incompetence and regurgitation are often used interchangeably in relation to valvular disease.

Mitral valve disease
There is a history of rheumatic fever in about half of the patients with mitral valve disease. Mitral stenosis is more common than mitral incompetence, although they may occur together.

Congestion of the lungs causes shortness of breath and tiredness; acute pulmonary oedema may occur. Atrial fibrillation is usually present and right heart failure gradually appears.

Aortic valve disease
Aortic valve disease may be due to congenital malformation,

endocarditis, syphilis or rheumatic heart disease. Stenosis or incompetence may occur.

Both aortic stenosis and incompetence result in enlargement (hypertrophy) of the muscle of the left ventricle. Left ventricular failure eventually occurs, followed by right heart failure. Breathlessness, tiredness and angina are the main symptoms.

Pulmonary and tricuspid valve disease

Tricuspid valve disease is usually due to rheumatic heart disease and is associated with mitral and aortic valve disease. Pulmonary valve disease is uncommon and is usually due to congenital malformation.

Right heart failure results from these conditions; back pressure is transmitted via the vena cava into the systemic circulation.

Medical and nursing intervention in valvular disease

Cardiac failure is treated (see page 76). Cardiac surgery may be performed and involves either valvotomy (dilation of the valve) or valve replacement. The types of valve in use are:

homografts — human tissue
heterografts — non-human tissue, e.g. pig valves
mechanical valves

Anticoagulant therapy is necessary for life following insertion of mechanical valves in order to prevent thrombus formation. There is an infection risk associated with this type of surgery.

Patients who are preparing to have cardiac surgery require careful explanation about the procedure and their postoperative care. It is helpful if they are able to meet a nurse from the intensive care unit who can help provide explanations and be a familiar face postoperatively.

Ischaemic heart disease

Ischaemic heart disease is caused by a reduction in the blood supply to the heart and is usually due to atherosclerosis of the coronary arteries. Fatty substances such as cholesterol are deposited in the walls of the arteries, gradually narrowing the lumen. This results in a reduction of the blood supply to the myocardium and the pain known as *angina* occurs.

A clot of blood (thrombus) may form on the atheromatous plaque and block the artery, drastically reducing the blood supply to the myocardium. Necrosis of the area of muscle served by the affected artery occurs; this is termed a *myocardial infarction.*

Coronary heart disease is a leading cause of death in males aged 35 to 65 years; the incidence in women is also increasing. It is a disease of Western countries. A number of risk factors have been implicated:

  higher levels of serum cholesterol and triglycerides
  smoking
  decreased physical activity
  stress
  hypertension
  diabetes

Angina pectoris

Angina is the pain resulting from inadequate blood supply to the myocardium. The causes are:

  atherosclerosis
  severe anaemia
  hypertension   } where the requirements of the
  aortic stenosis } myocardium are increased

Medical and nursing problems

Pain
— central chest pain
— may radiate to the arms, neck and jaw
— associated with:
    exercise
    emotion
    cold weather
    heavy meals
Anxiety
Tachycardia

Medical investigation and treatment

● Glyceryl trinitrate is given sublingually to relieve pain. This drug lowers the blood pressure and dilates the coronary arteries.

- An electrocardiogram (ECG) is performed at rest and during exercise. Cardiac catheterization and coronary angiography may be necessary in more severe cases.
- Slow-release glyceryl trinitrate is used as prophylaxis. This drug is swallowed. Other drugs which may be used include isosorbide dinitrate and nifedipine.
- Beta-receptor blocking drugs such as propranolol and metoprolol are used to reduce the rate and force of the heart beat and so reduce the oxygen demands of the myocardium.
- Surgery is used to treat severe angina. Coronary artery by-pass grafts using the saphenous vein are increasingly being performed with good results.

Nursing intervention
- The patient is encouraged to rest during an attack.
- In the longer term, the patient should modify his activity without becoming an invalid.
- Stress should be avoided.
- A low-fat diet is recommended and, if the patient is obese, weight should be reduced.
- The patient should stop smoking.

Myocardial infarction

A myocardial infarction occurs when the blood supply to an area of the myocardium becomes blocked. The resulting damage is irreversible.

Medical and nursing problems

Pain	Distress
— *severe* central chest pain	Sweating
— radiating to the neck, jaw and arms	Pallor
	Shock
— comes on when the patient is resting	Shortness of breath
	Fever
— often last for 30 minutes	Nausea
	Cardiac arrhythmias
Vomiting	

Forty per cent of patients who suffer a myocardial infarction will die from it.

Medical investigation and treatment

- Diamorphine (5–10 mg intravenously) is given to relieve pain and can be repeated every three to four hours. An anti-emetic should be given at the same time.
- Oxygen (24–28% via a Ventimask) is prescribed in order to improve the oxygen supply to the myocardium.
- An electrocardiogram (ECG) and chest X-ray are performed and blood is taken for cardiac enzymes.
- Cardiac monitoring is usually carried out.
- Indomethacin, an anti-inflammatory drug, may be used to relieve chest pain caused by inflammation of the pericardium (pericarditis).
- A diuretic drug, e.g. frusemide, may be used to reduce pulmonary oedema.
- Diazepam may be prescribed to relieve anxiety and to provide sedation.
- Arrhythmias are treated as follows:
    Sinus bradycardia:
        atropine
        isoprenaline
    Atrial fibrillation:
        digoxin
        DC electroconversion
    Heart block:
        atropine
        isoprenaline
        pacemaker
    Ventricular ectopics:
        lignocaine
    Ventricular fibrillation:
        DC electroconversion
        sodium bicarbonate

Nursing intervention

- Reassurance is given.
- The patient rests in bed in a comfortable position.

- Respiratory rate, apical and radial beats and blood pressure are observed at least hourly. Temperature is monitored four-hourly.
- A fluid intake and output chart is kept to detect fluid overload or dehydration.
- Salt intake is restricted.
- The patient is weighed daily after the first 48 hours.
- Careful explanation about all procedures and equipment is given. The nurse should be positive about the patient's future expectations.
- Fever occurs 24 to 48 hours after a myocardial infarction. The patient should be fanned and sponged as necessary.
- The patient is advised to rest in bed for the first 48 hours after the myocardial infarction. Thereafter he may gradually increase his activities, firstly sitting in a chair, then walking to the lavatory, and so on.
- Constipation is prevented by adding bran to foods and by giving a well-balanced diet.
- A commode is preferable to a bedpan in the first 48 hours.

Conclusion

Congestive cardiac failure may follow myocardial infarction and may sometimes be a cause of death. Other complications are rupture of the ventricle and cardiogenic shock.

A period of rehabilitation is necessary following myocardial infarction. Activity is gradually increased, and at four weeks the patient may walk outside, drive, and resume sexual intercourse. Smoking should cease, food intake should be controlled, and the patient should attempt to adopt a more relaxed attitude to living.

Cardiac arrest

Cardiac arrest is a sudden failure of the heart to supply an adequate circulation. The most common causes are:

myocardial infarction
electrolyte imbalance
anaesthesia
drowning
electrocution

The heart should be restarted within three minutes to prevent irreparable damage to the brain cells due to lack of oxygen.

Medical and nursing problems
Loss of consciousness
Absence of major pulse
Pallor and cyanosis
Cessation of breathing
Dilation of the pupils
Ventricular fibrillation or asystole on the ECG

Nursing intervention
- The lower third of the sternum is thumped with a clenched fist.
- External cardiac massage is commenced: the heel of one hand is placed over the lower third of the sternum, the heel of the other hand is placed over the first, and the sternum is depressed forcefully at a rate of about 60 times/minute.
- The airway is cleared by removing false teeth. The neck is extended and the jaw pulled forward in order to stop the tongue falling back. A plastic oral airway is inserted and mouth-to-mouth resuscitation is commenced at a rate of one breath to every five cardiac compressions.
- An Ambu bag may be used to ventilate the lungs.
- The nurse should be familiar with the cardiac arrest telephone number and with the whereabouts of the emergency equipment.
- Relatives are escorted to a quiet room away from the activity. They should be kept informed of all developments.

Medical treatment
- An endotracheal tube is inserted when the anaesthetist arrives.
- An intravenous infusion is set up; it is usually inserted into the subclavian or the external jugular vein.
- The following drugs may be used during a cardiac arrest:
    sodium bicarbonate, 8.4% infusion
    calcium chloride, 10%
    isoprenaline

    adrenaline
    anti-arrhythmic drugs after resuscitation
- DC electroconversion will be used if ventricular fibrillation is present. Everyone should stand well clear of the patient and bed to avoid getting an electric shock.

Heart failure

Left-sided heart failure

Failure of the left side of the heart may be the result of hypertension, aortic valve disease, myocardial infarction, mitral incompetence or mitral stenosis.

Medical and nursing problems
Breathlessness
— at rest
— on exertion
— when lying flat
Coughing
Frothy pink sputum
'Rattling' in the trachea
Cyanosis
Pallor
Cold, moist skin

The above signs and symptoms are due to pulmonary venous congestion causing accumulation of fluid in the alveoli of the lungs (pulmonary oedema).

Medical investigation and treatment
- A chest X-ray is performed, which shows congestion of the lungs and enlargement of the heart.
- Diamorphine may be prescribed to relieve dyspnoea by reducing anxiety, to cause peripheral venous dilation and to reduce the sensitivity of the respiratory centre to the reflex stimulation of the congested lungs.
- Oxygen is prescribed.
- A diuretic, e.g. frusemide, is given to reduce fluid and sodium

overload. Frusemide is commonly given intravenously in the acute stage.

- A bronchodilator, e.g. aminophylline or salbutamol, may also be prescribed to relieve bronchospasm.
- An intravenous line for measurement of central venous pressure may be inserted.

Nursing intervention

- The patient is assisted to sit in a comfortable, well-supported position in bed or in an upright armchair. This position improves chest expansion and decreases venous return.
- A sputum pot is provided and expectoration encouraged.
- A fluid input and output chart is kept to assess the effectiveness of the diuretic. The patient is weighed daily.
- Salt intake is restricted.
- Pulse, respiration and blood pressure are recorded every two to four hours.
- In severe pulmonary oedema, the central venous pressure may be recorded via a central line. The normal range is 4 to 8 cm. Lower readings indicate dehydration; higher readings indicate fluid overload.
- The patient rests in bed until his condition is improved.

Right-sided heart failure

Right-sided heart failure is usually secondary to left-sided heart failure. Other causes are myocardial infarction affecting the right ventricle, chronic pulmonary diseases, tricuspid and pulmonary valve stenosis, and pericarditis. In chronic pulmonary disease, back pressure is transmitted from the lungs to the pulmonary artery, affecting the right heart and then the systemic venous circulation.

Medical and nursing problems

Ankle oedema	Sacral oedema
Ascites	Pleural effusion
Anorexia	due to enlargement
Nausea	of the liver, stomach and
Vomiting	bowel

Engorgement of the jugular
veins
Confusion
— due to insufficient
oxygenation of
the brain

Reduction in urine output
— due to congestion of the
kidney
Pain
— due to oedema
Chest pain

Medical treatment

- Digoxin is given to improve cardiac output and to assist in the excretion of excess fluid. Nausea may occur as a side-effect of digoxin; toxicity is indicated by a very slow pulse with coupled beats.
- Diamorphine is prescribed to relieve chest pain.
- A diuretic, e.g. frusemide, is given as in left-sided heart failure.
- Oxygen may be required, especially if confusion is present.
- Anti-emetics, e.g. metoclopramide, may be used to relieve nausea.

Nursing intervention

- Temperature, pulse, respiration and blood pressure are recorded at least every six hours.
- Weight is recorded daily to monitor for the development of fluid retention.
- A fluid input and output chart should be kept if renal failure is suspected.
- The patient rests in bed or in a chair, sitting in an upright position.
- Leg and breathing exercises are encouraged to help prevent the formation of deep venous thrombosis (see page 84) and pneumonia.
- The legs are elevated to assist venous return.
- The patient's position is changed at least two-hourly. The skin is often taut and friable and this may predispose to the formation of pressure sores. A sheepskin may be useful.
- A bed cradle is used to relieve pressure on the oedematous legs.
- Cot sides may be required if the patient is confused, in order to protect him from injury.
- A light, well-presented diet is offered. It should be low in sodium.

● A commode is easier to use than a bedpan. Constipation is prevented by giving a well-balanced diet, high in roughage. Bran or mild aperients may be helpful.

Conclusion

Patients with heart failure are often very anxious and require much reassurance, support and explanation. The patient's mobility and independence are increased as soon as possible. Community support may be required on discharge from hospital.

Cor pulmonale

Cor pulmonale is right-sided heart failure secondary to chronic obstructive airways disease. Chronic bronchitis, emphysema and occupational lung disease will increase the workload of the right heart.

The patient will have a productive cough and severe dyspnoea in addition to the other symptoms of right-sided heart failure.

Heart block

Heart block occurs when the conducting system of the heart is impaired, resulting in failure of initiation or conduction of the electrical impulses which precede contraction of the cardiac muscle.

If there is complete block at the atrioventricular node in the conducting system of the heart then the ventricles will beat at a rate of 30 to 40/minute. This rate cannot maintain cardiac output and results in an inadequate blood supply to the brain, kidneys, and the coronary arteries. Stokes–Adams attacks are episodes of syncope caused by periods of ventricular standstill. The treatment of complete heart block is insertion of an artificial pacemaker. This is an electronic device that delivers an electrical stimulus to the heart through a pacing wire electrode, which is inserted in or on the right ventricle. A permanent pacemaker involves embedding the pulse generator into the subcutaneous tissue in the chest wall or upper abdominal wall. The battery will have to be changed every six to ten years.

Sub-acute bacterial endocarditis

Sub-acute bacterial endocarditis is inflammation of the endocardium caused by bacteria. It usually occurs in patients who have existing valvular disease, congenital heart defects or prosthetic valves. Vegetations of bacteria form on the valves.

The causative organism is most often *Streptococcus viridans,* which is found in infected teeth, gums and tonsils. *Streptococcus viridans* may particularly be released into the bloodstream after dental extractions.

Medical and nursing problems

Fever
Tiredness
— due to anaemia
Anorexia
Malaise
Weight loss
Splinter haemorrhages
  under the nails
Petechial haemorrhages
  into the skin
Painful hard lumps
  on fingers and toes
  (Osler's nodes)
Haematuria
Raised white cell
  count
Raised erythocyte
  sedimentation rate
  (ESR)
Enlarged spleen

Medical investigation and treatment
- Blood cultures are taken and the causative organism is identified.
- Antibiotic therapy is commenced intravenously. Benzyl-penicillin is most commonly used and large doses are given for several weeks. Oral antibiotic therapy is started when the temperature falls.

Nursing intervention
- The patient is advised to rest in bed, only getting up to use the commode.
- Temperature, pulse and respiration are recorded four times daily, and the blood pressure taken at least once a day.
- Pressure area care and mouth care are required, and constipation is prevented.
- Mobilization is commenced when the fever has resolved.

Conclusion

There is a risk of embolism from the vegetations on the endocardium of the valves; hemiplegia, renal failure, loss of vision, or ischaemia of a limb may result. Severe heart failure may occur.

Prevention of endocarditis is essential. Every patient with valvular disease or congenital heart disease should receive prophylactic antibiotics, usually penicillin, before and after dental treatment. Respiratory tract infections should be treated promptly.

Pericarditis

Pericarditis is inflammation of the pericardium. It may occur after acute myocardial infarction, or during rheumatic fever or tuberculosis. It may also occur as a complication of other disorders, e.g. uraemia or connective tissue disorders.

Chest pain is usually present, a friction 'rub' is heard on auscultation, and a chest X-ray may show a collection of fluid in the pericardial sac. Fever is usually present.

The underlying cause is treated. Indomethacin, an anti-inflammatory drug, is useful in the relief of pain.

Hypertension

Raised blood pressure (hypertension) may be defined as a diastolic blood pressure persistently above 90 mmHg. Blood pressure increases with age in Western societies.

Hypertension may be primary (essential) or secondary. Primary hypertension accounts for 90% of all cases. The cause is unknown, although obesity, stress and a familial tendency may be contributory factors. The major blood vessels become sclerosed and narrowed.

Secondary hypertension accounts for the remaining 10% of patients. The most common causes are:

Renal disease

Endocrine disease, e.g. phaeochromocytoma, Cushing's disease

Cardiovascular disease, e.g. coarctation of the aorta

Hormone therapy, e.g. oral contraceptives, steroids

Drug therapy, e.g. some antidepressants

Other causes, e.g. pregnancy, raised intracranial pressure

Medical and nursing problems

Hypertension may produce
no symptoms
Headache
Vomiting
Memory impairment
Blood pressure consistently
higher than 90 mm Hg
diastolic
Shortness of breath and
angina
— due to increased workload
on the heart

Proteinuria
— due to renal impairment
— chronic renal failure
may result
Visual disturbances
— retinal haemorrhages
— oedema of the
optic disc
(papilloedema)

Medical investigation and treatment

● Blood is taken for estimation of urea and electrolytes. Increased
levels may indicate renal impairment.
● An intravenous urogram (see page 180) is performed.
● Diuretics are very useful for the more elderly patients.
Cyclopenthiazide with potassium (Navidrex-K) and bendro-
fluazide are commonly used.
● Common antihypertensive drugs include:
beta-blockers, e.g. propranolol
alpha-blockers, e.g. labetalol
vasodilators, e.g. hydralazine, prazosin
others, e.g. methyldopa, captopril
Postural hypotension may occur as a side effect of some of these
drugs.
● A 24-hour urine collection for vanillylmandelic acid (VMA) is
normally performed in order to detect the presence of a rare
tumour of the adrenal glands — a phaeochromocytoma —
which may cause hypertension. The patient should not eat
foods containing vanilla throughout the duration of this test.

Nursing intervention

● The urine is tested for blood and protein.
● The blood pressure is recorded at least six-hourly, with the
patient lying and standing.

- Careful explanation is required in order that compliancy with drug therapy is satisfactory.
- Advice is given concerning restriction of salt and animal fat in the diet.
- The obese patient may require a low-calorie diet.
- Stress should be avoided and smoking should cease.

Complications of hypertension

Hypertension, if inadequately treated, may predispose to myocardial infarction, congestive cardiac failure, end stage renal failure, cerebrovascular accident and loss of vision.

Malignant hypertension is said to occur when there is severe hypertension, papilloedema, retinal haemmorhages and renal failure.

Peripheral vascular disease

Peripheral vascular disease results in reduced circulation to the limbs causing lack of oxygen and nutrients in the tissues.

The most common cause is atherosclerosis. This condition usually affects people over the age of 50, and is more common in men. Diabetics are particularly prone to peripheral vascular disease.

Medical and nursing problems

Intermittent claudication
— pain on exercise which ceases with rest
Cold extremities
Ulceration
Gangrene

Medical investigation and treatment

- Arteriography may be performed to show the extent of damage to the arteries.
- Surgical procedures may sometimes be indicated.
- Analgesia is prescribed to relieve pain.
- A sedative may be required at night if insomnia is present.

Nursing intervention
- The obese patient is given dietary advice.
- Animal fats are restricted and smoking should cease.
- Good control of diabetes is essential.
- The patient is advised to visit a chiropodist regularly, to avoid injury to the feet, and to have infections treated promptly.
- Well-fitting shoes and socks are essential.
- Extremities of heat and cold should be avoided.

Deep venous thrombosis

Deep venous thrombosis (DVT) is a solid clot of blood occurring in the deep veins of the leg. Forty per cent of such clots are bilateral. The thrombosis may extend along the full length of the blood vessel.

Predisposing factors to the formation of deep venous thrombosis are:

Stasis
— reduced cardiac output
— lack of muscular activity
— varicose veins
— decreased venous return
Damage to the vessel wall
— external pressures, e.g. plasters, pillows
— trauma

— diseases of the vessel, e.g. atheroma
Increased viscosity of the blood
— contraceptive pill
— pregnancy
— polycythaemia
— after surgery, shock, childbirth

Medical and nursing problems

Calf pain
— worse on dorsiflexion of the foot (Homan's sign)
Tenderness of the calf

Oedema of calf or foot
Inflammation
— local redness
— increased heat

Medical investigation and treatment
- Ultrasound or phlebography may be used in the diagnosis of deep vein thrombosis.
- Anticoagulant therapy is started immediately. Heparin acts rapidly and is used for the first two to three days. It may be given intravenously or subcutaneously. Warfarin, an oral anticoagulant, takes longer to act. A 'loading' dose is given 24

to 48 hours before the heparin is stopped. Thereafter a daily dose of warfarin is given.
- Blood is taken daily to determine the prothrombin time ratio (PTR), which indicates how long the blood takes to clot; from this result the dose of warfarin needed is decided.

Nursing intervention
- The patient is encouraged to rest in bed for a few days.
- Anti-embolism stockings are worn.
- The foot of the bed is elevated to promote venous return, and a bed cradle is used to relieve the pressure of the bed clothes.
- The patient is advised to drink at least two litres of fluid/day to prevent increased viscosity of the blood.
- Constipation is avoided by supplementing the diet with bran, fruit and vegetables.
- Deep breathing exercises are performed.
- After a few days' rest, the patient is allowed to get up and resume normal activities.
- Urine is tested daily for blood and the patient is observed for signs of bruising, as there is a risk of haemorrhage with anticoagulation.

Prevention
Deep breathing exercises help venous blood to return to the heart. Leg exercises utilize the muscular pump to squeeze blood upwards. Both these types of exercises should be performed by all patients who are at risk of developing a deep venous thrombosis. Ideally they should be performed for five minutes of each hour. Patients who are unable to perform these exercises alone should be assisted by nursing staff, physiotherapists and relatives.

Anti-embolic stockings should be worn by high risk patients. Subcutaneous heparin is sometimes given prophylactically, e.g. prior to surgery.

Pulmonary embolus

Pulmonary embolus occurs when a portion of thrombus from a systemic vein is detached and enters the circulation. It may lodge in a pulmonary artery and cause sudden death. There is a 50% mortality rate associated with this condition.

Severe chest pain, breathlessness, cyanosis and shock may occur with massive embolism, whilst symptoms may be absent with small emboli.

An electrocardiogram and lung scan are performed. Relief of pain is important; morphine may be necessary. Oxygen is given at four litres/minute via an MC mask. The treatment of pulmonary embolus is the same as that for deep venous thrombosis.

Further reading

Hubner, P. (1980) *Nurses' Guide to Cardiac Monitoring,* 3rd edition. London: Baillière Tindall.
Julian, D.Y. (1983) *Cardiology,* 4th edition. London: Baillière Tindall.
Thompson, D. (1982) *Cardiac Nursing* London: Baillière Tindall.

6
Respiratory Nursing

The respiratory system allows oxygen to be absorbed into the blood and carbon dioxide to be excreted. During inspiration atmospheric air is sucked in through the nose, pharynx, larynx, trachea, bronchi, bronchioles and alveolar ducts to reach the alveoli (Figure 21). Oxygen then passes from the alveoli into the capillary blood, and carbon dioxide passes from the blood into the alveoli to be expired (Figure 22). Oxygenated blood is carried by the circulatory system to all the tissues in the body.

The following terms are used to describe abnormal functions of the respiratory system:

Dyspnoea — difficulty in breathing

Apnoea — temporary cessation of breathing

Orthopnoea — difficulty in breathing unless in an upright position

Hypoxia — reduced oxygen supply to the tissues

Cyanosis — blue discoloration of the skin or mucous membranes caused by imperfect oxygenation of the blood

Nursing assessment of the patient with respiratory disease

The nurse who admits a patient suffering from a respiratory disorder will usually identify the first problem as breathlessness. This can result from any obstruction to breathing, especially excessive secretions, foreign bodies, malignancy, or spasm and oedema of the small air passages. A pneumothorax, injuries of the chest wall, or damage to the respiratory centre can also cause an increase in the respiratory rate. The breathless patient will also be anxious and tired. His fear may increase his respiratory rate further.

Sputum is formed as a result of infection, inflammation or congestion. The nurse should observe the colour, consistency and quantity of the sputum. Purulent sputum consists mainly of pus; mucoid sputum is clear and slightly sticky. Haemoptysis is blood-stained sputum. Frothy sputum is usually due to pulmonary oedema.

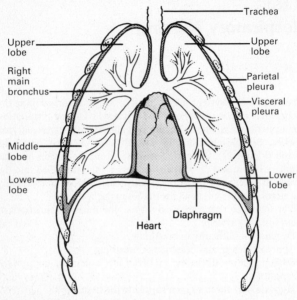

Figure 21. The respiratory tract.

Cough in respiratory disorders may be dry and irritating, or productive. A dry cough can be exhausting, particularly at night.

Chest pain may be due to tracheitis, when it is worse on coughing, or inflammation of the pleura, when it is greatest on inspiration.

Cyanosis indicates that there is insufficient oxygenation of the blood. It is a sign of respiratory failure.

Oxygen therapy

Hypoxia is a common consequence of respiratory disease and oxygen therapy is frequently prescribed.

Methods of administration are:

1   *Ventimask* (Figure 23): used when an accurate percentage of oxygen is required, especially in chronic respiratory disease. These masks can deliver 24%, 28% or 35% oxygen. They do not allow rebreathing of carbon dioxide.

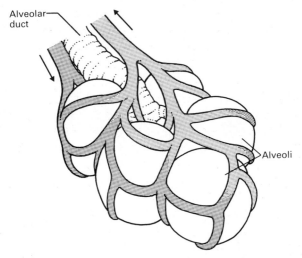

Figure 22. The alveoli and capillary network.

2 *MC mask or Hudson mask* (Figure 24): used when high concentrations of oxygen are required, e.g. 35 to 65%. Rebreathing of carbon dioxide occurs.

3 *Nasal cannulae* (Figure 25): these allow the patient to eat and drink normally, and to communicate easily. The concentration of oxygen may vary.

4 *Oxygen tents:* used for young children.

5 *Head boxes:* useful for infants and young children.

6 *Ventilators:* can be operated with air or oxygen. A range of concentrations can be used.

The mouth and nose can become very dry during oxygen therapy. Fluids are encouraged and mouth care performed. These patients often appreciate ice to suck. Humidification is necessary with high concentrations of oxygen.

In chronic obstructive airways disease, sensitivity of the respiratory centre to carbon dioxide is impaired and the patient relies on the hypoxic drive to maintain respiration. If too high a concentration of oxygen is given, carbon dioxide retention will occur and respiration will be depressed. The nurse should observe these patients continuously for signs of respiratory depression.

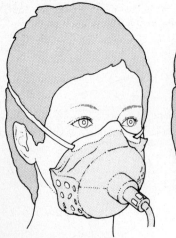

Figure 23. A Ventimask.

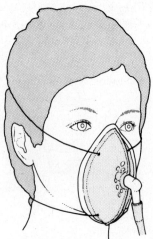

Figure 24. A MC mask or Hudson mask.

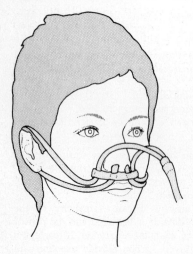

Figure 25. Nasal cannulae.

Oxygen in excess is toxic to the lining of the bronchi and alveoli, eventually leading to gross stiffness of the lungs and hypoxia.

Oxygen supports combustion, therefore smoking should be prohibited in an area where oxygen is being used.

Investigations

Lung function tests
Vital capacity is the largest volume of air which can be expelled from the lungs after full inspiration. It measures loss of lung volume.

Peak expiratory flow rate (PEFR) is the maximum flow, in litres/minute, at the beginning of forced expiration from full inspiration. It is measured using a peak flow meter, and measures airflow obstruction.

Arterial blood gases measure gas transfer from the air to the blood.

Radiography
All respiratory patients will have an X-ray of the chest. Tomograms illustrate the depth of lesions in the lung. Screening can be used to determine the position and function of the diaphragm.

A bronchogram is the introduction of dye into the lungs to outline the walls of the bronchi. Radioisotope scanning may be performed, and is of special value when pulmonary emboli are suspected.

Bronchoscopy
A flexible fibreoptic bronchoscope is used to inspect the trachea and larger bronchi (Figure 26). Tissue can be removed (a biopsy) for examination. This procedure is usually performed under local anaesthesia. A rigid bronchoscope is used for removal of foreign bodies or copious secretions.

After bronchoscopy the patient must have nothing to eat or drink until the cough reflex has returned.

Laryngoscopy
Indirect laryngoscopy is inspection of the larynx using a small

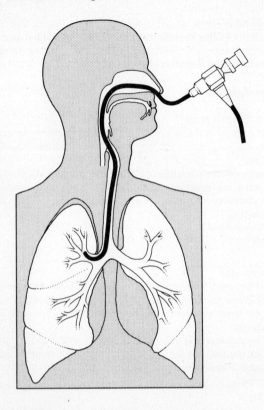

Figure 26. Fibreoptic bronchoscopy.

mirror placed at the back of the mouth. Direct laryngoscopy is inspection of the larynx using a laryngoscope.

Mediastinoscopy

Mediastinoscopy is inspection of the mediastinum using a fibreoptic endoscope through a small incision in the chest wall. Enlarged lymph nodes can be biopsied.

Pleural aspiration

Fluid is aspirated from the pleural cavity using a large-bore needle and syringe. This procedure is performed under local anaesthesia. The specimen of fluid is sent to the laboratory for bacteriological and cytological tests.

The nurse should observe the patient's respiratory rate and sputum after the investigation.

A pleural biopsy is sometimes taken at the same time as a pleural aspiration; for this an Abraham's pleural punch is used.

Sputum

Sputum specimens may be sent to the laboratory for bacteriological or cytological examination.

Infections of the respiratory system

Acute bronchitis

Bronchitis is defined as inflammation of the mucous membranes of the bronchial tree.

Causes

Acute bronchitis is usually caused by bacteria such as *Streptococcus pneumoniae* and *Haemophilus influenzae.* It can be a complication of the common cold, influenza, measles, or whooping cough. Patients who have chronic bronchitis are very prone to episodes of acute bronchitis.

Acute bronchitis is more common in the winter months when the patient may be exposed to damp, cold or foggy conditions. Cigarette smoking may also predispose to acute bronchitis.

Medical and nursing problems
Cough
— dry and irritating at first
— productive later
Chest pain
— retrosternal pain
— due to tracheitis

Sputum
— mucopurulent
— sometimes streaked with blood
Fever
— low-grade pyrexia
In severe cases the temperature may rise to 38–39°C and dyspnoea and cyanosis may be present.

Medical investigation and treatment
- Sputum specimens are taken for microbiological examination.
- Antibiotic treatment, e.g. amoxicillin, is commenced.
- Aspirin may help to relieve pain and reduce the high fever.
- Oxygen and bronchodilator drugs are rarely needed in acute uncomplicated bronchitis.

Nursing intervention
- If the patient is breathless, he is assisted to sit upright in bed, with his back well supported.
- Reassurance and explanation of treatment is essential to relieve anxiety, which in turn will help reduce a fast respiratory rate.
- Temperature, pulse and respiratory rate are recorded at least six-hourly. The nurse should be alert to signs of exhaustion and respiratory depression.
- The patient's colour is observed for signs of cyanosis.
- The physiotherapist and nurse can assist and encourage the patient to cough in order to expectorate his sputum.
- A good fluid intake of two or three litres/day will decrease the viscosity of the sputum and so aid expectoration.

Conclusion
The patient should be advised to stop smoking. Poor housing conditions may need to be investigated by the medical social worker.

Pneumonia

Pneumonia is inflammation of the lung. Exudates of fluid, protein and red blood cells cause consolidation of the inflamed area. There are two main groups:

1 *Lobar pneumonia* — an acute primary infection occurring in a previously healthy respiratory tract. The whole of a lobe of the lung becomes consolidated.

2 *Bronchopneumonia* — infected material is aspirated from the upper respiratory tract. Patches of inflammation are scattered in one lobe, several lobes, or over both lungs. Bronchopneumonia commonly occurs secondary to other conditions such as chronic bronchitis or carcinoma of the bronchus.

Causes

Pneumonia is usually caused by bacteria. Common organisms causing lobar pneumonia are *Streptococcus pneumoniae* (pneumococcus), *Streptococcus pyogenes*, *Klebsiella pneumoniae* and *Mycoplasma pneumoniae*. Viruses may also be responsible for lobar pneumonias.

Common organisms causing bronchopneumonia are *Streptococcus pneumoniae*, *Staphylococcus aureus* and *Haemophilus influenzae*.

People who are susceptible to pneumonia are those suffering from:

Viral infections
— influenza
— measles
— chickenpox
Chronic obstructive airways disease
Bronchial obstruction
— tumours
— foreign bodies
— retention of secretions (especially following anaesthesia)
Aspiration
— unconsciousness
— oesophageal fistula
— motor neurone disease
Impaired resistance
— steroid or cytotoxic therapy
— elderly
— malnutrition
— very young
— diabetes mellitus
— chronic renal failure

Medical and nursing problems
Fever
— 38–40°C
— causes rigors
Systemic disturbances
— vomiting
Confusion
— especially in the elderly
— due to hypoxia
Respiratory symptoms
— dyspnoea
— rapid respiration rate
— pleuritic chest pain
— cough
— cyanosis
— sputum
Cardiovascular symptoms
— tachycardia
— atrial fibrillation and heart failure in the very young and old
— hypotension due to dehydration and infection
Herpes simplex
— around the mouth and lips
— in lobar pneumonia

In lobar pneumonia, the patient may expectorate rusty coloured sputum; the colour is due to altered blood. In bronchopneumonia, sputum may be scanty at first and purulent later. Haemoptysis often occurs.

Medical investigation and treatment
- Oxygen therapy may be prescribed if the patient is hypoxic.
- A sputum specimen is taken for microbiological examination.
- Antibiotics are prescribed. These may be given orally or intravenously.
- Intravenous fluids may be necessary if severe dehydration is present.
- Mild analgesics, e.g. paracetamol or aspirin, are prescribed to relieve chest pain.
- Bronchodilator drugs, e.g. salbutamol, are given in more severe cases.

Nursing intervention
- Rest is essential. The patient is often most comfortable when sitting upright, but it may be preferable to nurse the patient on his side to facilitate the removal of secretions from the bases of the lungs.
- Respiratory rate, level of consciousness and colour are closely observed, particularly if oxygen therapy is being used (see page 88).
- Temperature and pulse are recorded six-hourly. Fanning is helpful when the temperature rises above 38°C.
- A fluid intake of two to three litres/day is necessary to prevent dehydration due to sweating and the rapid respiratory rate.
- The patient is encouraged to cough and expectorate.
- Confusion may be present due to hypoxia, and cot sides may be required to prevent injury.
- If the patient cannot tolerate an oxygen mask, nasal cannulae should be considered as an alternative.
- Attention to hygiene, particularly mouth care, is necessary.
- The elderly patient will be very susceptible to skin breakdown and therefore the patient's position should be changed at least two-hourly.
- High-calorie, high-protein drinks are often appreciated by a patient who is unable to manage a solid diet.

Advice on discharge
Pneumonia can be debilitating, therefore the patient should be advised to rest. Elderly patients may require a long stay in hospital before they are fully recovered.

Conclusion
There is a high mortality rate in bronchopneumonia, especially in the very young and the old. Early treatment of respiratory infections is essential.

Pulmonary tuberculosis

Pulmonary tuberculosis is a disease caused by the micro-organism *Mycobacterium tuberculosis*. The human type of the mycobacterium is most commonly responsible for the disease in man. Bovine tuberculosis has been eradicated in the United Kingdom as a result of the pasteurization of milk and the veterinary inspection of cattle.

Most tuberculosis infections are due to the inhalation of air containing the tubercle bacilli, coughed up by an infectious person.

An area of inflammation occurs in the alveoli (primary focus), and the lymph nodes in the hilum of the lung enlarge. This infection usually resolves unnoticed. Failure to resolve will result in an area of caseation (cheese-like consistency). Fibrosis and calcification may occur, resulting in lung cavities. Pleural effusion, haemoptysis and pneumothorax may result.

Miliary tuberculosis occurs when the tubercle bacilli spread into the bloodstream. Tuberculosis of bones, joints and the genito-urinary tract may occur. Tuberculosis meningitis may also accompany this condition.

Predisposing factors

Tuberculosis is most commonly seen in the underdeveloped countries. There is a high incidence among the Asian immigrants in Great Britain. Tuberculosis is associated with overcrowded housing, poor nutrition, and alcoholism. It is more common in males over the age of 45 years.

Patients with the following conditions are susceptible to tuberculosis:
diabetes
steroid or immunosuppressive therapy
congenital heart disease
gastrectomy

Medical and nursing problems

Uncomplicated primary infection may be symptomless	Pleuritic pain
	Hoarseness
	— due to laryngitis
Fever	Cough
— night sweats	— usually productive
Anorexia and weight loss	— haemoptysis
Anaemia	Dyspnoea

Medical investigation and treatment

● Sputum specimens are taken in order to identify the 'acid fast' tubercle bacilli.

- The patient is isolated if acid fast bacilli are present. Isolation is discontinued after three to five days of drug treatment as the risk of infection is then minimal.
- Vitamin supplements are prescribed in order to improve the patient's nutritional state.
- Treatment with anti-tuberculous drugs can last 18 months to two years. Three anti-tuberculous drugs are given at first; this is known as 'triple therapy'. Three drugs are used as resistance can quickly develop if only one is used. The most commonly used drugs are:

   Rifampicin (400–600 mg daily)
   — colours the urine red
   Isoniazid (200–300 mg daily)
   — may cause peripheral neuritis
   — pyridoxine (vitamin B_6) 10 mg often given
      prophylactically
   Ethambutol (15 mg/kg daily)
   — may cause optic neuritis

- In underdeveloped countries streptomycin and isoniazid are used on two days/week.

Nursing intervention
- Reassurance and careful explanation is given.
- Great care is taken when disposing of infected sputum.
- Masks are worn by all personnel entering the isolation room, and gloves are worn when sputum is handled. The patient has his own crockery inside the room.
- A good nutritional state is necessary to aid recovery. Milk and other high protein supplements are encouraged.
- The urine is tested daily for bilirubin and urobilinogen because of the risk of liver damage from the anti-tuberculous drugs.
- Gloves are worn when administering intramuscular streptomycin as skin rashes are liable to occur.
- Patients with tuberculosis may present with symptoms of pneumonia and will then require the relevant nursing care (see page 97).

Advice on discharge
The patient is discharged from hospital when his sputum is no longer infectious. He is advised to comply with his drug therapy and to attend his outpatient appointment.

Conclusion

Tuberculosis should be notified to the Community Physician. Contacts will then be screened and, if necessary, treated. Prevention of tuberculosis is essential.

Tuberculin testing is carried out on all school children in Great Britain, and BCG vaccination is given as necessary. Regular chest radiography shold be performed on susceptible groups, and socio-economic conditions should be improved wherever possible.

Chronic obstructive airways disease

Chronic bronchitis and emphysema often coexist and are grouped together under the term 'chronic obstructive airways disease'.

Chronic bronchitis is chronic inflammation of the lung due to long-term exposure of the broncial mucosa to irritants.

Emphysema is the enlargement of the alveoli and the destruction of their walls. The lungs become overdistended and lose their normal elasticity. It is frequently associated with chronic bronchitis.

Chronic obstructive airways disease is more common in middle-aged and elderly men.

Causes

The common irritants which cause chronic bronchitis are tobacco smoke, dust, fumes and smoke. Infection aggravates the condition and is usually due to the bacteria *Streptococcus pneumoniae* or *Haemophilus influenzae.*

This condition is usually worse during the winter months, especially after exposure to dampness, fog, or a change in temperature.

Medical and nursing problems
Cough
— repeated attacks of a productive 'winter cough'
— usually worse in the morning
Sputum
— sometimes scanty, mucoid and tenacious
— sometimes copious and watery

— purulent if bacterial infection is present
Dyspnoea
— worse on exertion
— caused by airways obstruction
— aggravated by infection and mucosal oedema
Barrel-shaped, rigid chest (in emphysema)
Cyanosis
— worse on exertion
Peripheral oedema
— due to right-sided heart failure (cor pulmonale)

Medical investigation and treatment
- Oxygen at 24–28% via a Ventimask is prescribed.
- Blood gases are taken to monitor oxygen requirements.
- Sputum specimens are taken for microbiological examination.
- Antibiotics, e.g. amoxycillin, are used to treat the chest infection.
- Bronchodilator drugs, e.g. salbutamol, can be given by inhalation, in tablet form or intravenously. Aminophylline, another bronchodilator, is especially useful when given in suppository form prior to the patient settling for the night.
- Diuretics, e.g. frusemide, will reduce peripheral oedema.
- Hypnotics and sedatives are avoided as they may lead to respiratory depression.

Nursing intervention
- The patient is assisted to sit upright in bed or in a high-backed comfortable chair. He will be breathless even at rest.
- Reassurance and explanation are given.
- Respiratory rate, level of consciousness and colour should be observed carefully whilst the patient is receiving oxygen (see page 88).
- Temperature and pulse are recorded at least six-hourly.
- A fluid intake of two to three litres/24 hours is encouraged to aid expectoration of sputum.
- The patient will require intensive physiotherapy. The nurse can assist the patient to cough and expectorate.
- Weight is recorded daily in order to monitor the effect of any diuretics used.

- Maintenance of personal hygiene is essential. Mouthwashes should be given frequently as the mouth may be dry as a result of oxygen therapy.
- Many patients with chronic bronchitis are disabled and therefore susceptible to skin breakdown. The patient's position should be changed at least two-hourly.

Advice on discharge

The patient should be advised to avoid irritants such as smoke, dust or fumes. He may need to change his occupation to achieve this. Respiratory infections should be treated promptly.

Conclusion

Chronic obstructive airways disease can be very disabling. Premature retirement may be necessary resulting in socio-economic problems. The patient may eventually become housebound, often relying on oxygen to move from room to room. He may need the support of community services such as a home help and meals-on-wheels. Britain has the highest mortality rate from bronchitis.

Bronchiectasis

Bronchiectasis is chronic dilation of the bronchi and bronchioles with impaired drainage of bronchial secretions. There is persistent infection in the affected lobe or segment. The incidence of this condition has fallen as a result of effective antibiotic therapy.

Causes

Bronchial obstruction
— mucous plugs
— tumours
— foreign bodies
Congenital disorders
Cystic fibrosis
— obstruction by viscid sputum

Medical and nursing problems

Symptoms usually begin in childhood.

Chronic cough
Sputum
— purulent and copious
— worse in the morning
— haemoptysis common
Dyspnoea
— only present when bronchiectasis is bilateral
Sinusitis
Systemic symptoms
— weight loss and anorexia
— fever
Finger clubbing

Medical investigation and treatment
- Sputum specimens are taken for microbiological culture and sensitivity.
- Infections are treated promptly with antibiotics.
- Surgical intervention, e.g. removal of a lobe of the lung, may be necessary.

Nursing intervention
- Postural drainage of the affected lobe is essential, and a member of the family should be taught to percuss the chest.
- Coughing and deep breathing exercises are encouraged, particularly on rising in the morning.
- The breathless patient may prefer to sit upright in bed in order to sleep.
- A good fluid intake is essential in order to reduce the viscosity of the sputum and so aid expectoration.
- A high-protein, high-calorie diet is given.

Conclusion
Antibiotic therapy has improved the prognosis, and complications such as pneumonia are now rare.

Asthma

Bronchial asthma is a temporary narrowing of the bronchi by muscle spasm and mucosal oedema. Air becomes trapped in the alveoli. It is characterized by paroxysms of dyspnoea and wheezing.

Types of asthma

1 *Extrinsic asthma* occurs in people who are allergic to common allergens, including house dust, mites, grass pollen, fur and feathers. There is usually a family history of allergic disease, especially eczema and hayfever. These individuals are described as being 'atopic'.

2 *Intrinsic asthma* occurs in non-atopic individuals in later life. There is no obvious allergic factor.

The symptoms of asthma can be precipitated by exposure to dust, tobacco smoke, fumes, infection and stress.

Medical and nursing problems

Dyspnoea
— paroxysms of dyspnoea and wheezing
— wheeze is more pronounced on expiration
— accessory muscles are used to aid expiration
— exhaustion can lead to respiratory failure
Cyanosis
— the face becomes congested
— extremities are cyanosed
Tachycardia
— present in severe attacks
Sputum
— scanty at first
— sometimes viscid
Stress
Status asthmaticus
— severe, worsening asthma
— eventually leads to:
    exhausation and inability to cough
    cyanosis
    disturbances of consciousness
    respiratory failure

Medical investigation and treatment

- Oxygen is prescribed, and usually administered via an MC mask.
- Salbutamol, a bronchodilator, can be given by inhaler or nebulizer. In more severe cases, another bronchodilator, aminophylline (250–500 mg) can be given intravenously.

- Steroids are given to reduce oedema of the mucosa, e.g. hydrocortisone (100–200 mg six-hourly). The dose of steroid is reduced slowly when the patient's condition has stabilized.
- If the patient fails to respond to this treatment he may require assisted ventilation.
- Antibiotics, e.g. amoxicillin, are used to treat the underlying respiratory infection. These may be given orally or intravenously.
- Dehydration is corrected using intravenous fluids.
- Sputum specimens are taken for microbiological examination.
- Hypnotics and sedatives are avoided as they may lead to respiratory depression.
- Blood gases are taken in order to monitor oxygen requirements.

Nursing intervention
- The breathless, anxious patient is assisted to sit upright in bed and reassurance is given.
- Respiratory rate, level of consciousness and colour are closely observed whilst the patient is receiving oxygen (see page 88).
- Temperature, pulse and blood pressure are monitored half-hourly to four-hourly, depending on the severity of the attack.
- Intensive physiotherapy is given to aid expectoration of the viscid sputum.
- Peak flow readings are taken in order to monitor the response to the bronchodilator drugs.
- A good fluid intake of two to three litres/24 hours will decrease the viscosity of the sputum and so aid expectoration.
- Urine is tested each day for sugar because of the risk of steroid-induced diabetes.

Advice on discharge
The patient is advised to avoid causative allergens. Respiratory infections should be treated promptly. Stressful situations should be avoided as they may precipitate an attack.

Salbutamol given using an inhaler or Rotacaps and a Rotahaler can be used by the patient during an asthmatic attack. Steroids can be given in the form of a beclomethasone inhaler. Sodium cromoglycate (Intal), given via an inhaler, prevents release of agents which cause bronchoconstriction and is used prophylactically.

Conclusion
The causative allergens can be identified by patch tests and should then be avoided if possible. It is essential to live as normal a life as possible; relatives can often become very protective towards a child with asthma. Many children with asthma will be symptom-free by the age of 15 years.

Carcinoma of the bronchus

Carcinoma of the bronchus is the most common primary neoplasm in men in Britain. It is a disease of middle and old age. The incidence among women is increasing.

Causes
The incidence of bronchial carcinoma is higher in cigarette smokers and those living in urban areas.

Workers who are exposed to asbestos, nickel and radioactive substances have an increased risk of bronchial carcinoma.

Medical and nursing problems

Cough	Systemic disturbances
Sputum	— weight loss
— sometimes bloodstained	— anorexia
— sometimes purulent	— weakness
because of secondary	— dysphagia
infection	— hoarseness
Chest pain	Symptoms due to metastatic
Breathlessness	deposits
— rarely disabling	— e.g. bone pain or hemiplegia

Medical investigation and treatment
- Analgesia is prescribed to relieve pain. The type of analgesic used will depend upon the severity of the pain.
- Carcinoma of the bronchus can be treated by surgery, radiotherapy, chemotherapy, or a combination of these.
- Surgical treatment consists of a lobectomy (removal of a lobe) or pneumonectomy (removal of a lung).

- Radiotherapy can be used to treat a primary tumour or can be used palliatively to treat bone pain, severe haemoptysis or breathlessness. Anti-emetics, e.g. prochlorperazine (5 mg), may be required to prevent nausea and vomiting associated with the radiotherapy.
- Chemotherapy is occasionally used in the treatment of carcinoma of the bronchus. Nausea, vomiting and alopecia may occur as side-effects. Anti-emetics are given to relieve nausea and vomiting.

Nursing intervention
- The patient with carcinoma of the bronchus will probably be anxious and frightened. Thorough explanations of the investigations and types of treatment are essential.
- Analgesia is given regularly, e.g. three-hourly, to prevent pain.
- Anti-emetics are more effective if given prior to radiotherapy or chemotherapy.
- The nurse should encourage small, appetizing meals and give frequent mouth care.
- Skin reactions to radiotherapy can occur and the patient should avoid wetting the area marked for treatment.

Conclusion
The prognosis of carcinoma of the bronchus is poor. Of patients who have had surgery, 25 to 30% survive five years; however, surgery is only feasible for 25% of patients.

The patient and his family will need much support from their general practitioner, district nurse and social worker. The hospice movement is expanding, and in many areas a terminal care support team is available to look after these patients in their own homes.

The risk of developing carcinoma of the bronchus can be reduced by a reduction in cigarette smoking. Protective clothing should be worn by workers who are exposed to carcinogenic substances.

Occupational lung diseases

The most common occupational lung diseases are those caused by inhalation of mineral dusts (pneumoconiosis). Fibrosis of the lung can occur, resulting in progressive breathlessness, respiratory failure and cardiac failure. The most common types of pneumoconiosis are:

   coal worker's pneumoconiosis
   silicosis
   asbestosis

Silicosis can predispose to pulmonary tuberculosis. Asbestosis can predispose to malignant disease of the pleura and peritoneum.

The Department of Health and Social Security provide compensation for those workers affected by occupational lung diseases. Prevention, however, is very important. Industries are obliged by law to ensure their workers use respirators where necessary. Adequate ventilation and damping down of dust is essential.

Disorders of the pleura

Pneumothorax

A pneumothorax is a collection of air in the pleural space causing collapse of the associated lung.

Causes
A spontaneous pneumothorax occurs when a sac of air in the lung (a bulla) ruptures through the surface of the visceral pleura, allowing air to escape into the pleural space. Spontaneous pneumothorax mainly occurs in healthy people, especially tall young men, and is often recurrent. Patients with chronic bronchitis and emphysema are also susceptible due to the large air sacs that may develop in the lungs in these conditions.

A pneumothorax can also be caused by penetrating wounds of the chest wall and by rib fractures. If blood is also present in the pleural space, the condition is known as a haemopneumothorax.

Types
1   Closed pneumothorax (Figure 27). The hole between the lung and the pleural space (marked A on Figure 27) closes off and the air in the pleural cavity is gradually absorbed, allowing the lung to re-expand.

2   Open pneumothorax (Figure 28). The hole between the lung

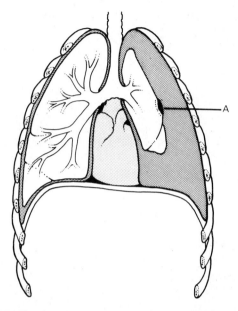

Figure 27. Closed pneumothorax.

and the pleural space remains open and the lung thus remains deflated. Sometimes a direct communication between the bronchus and the pleural space can develop; this is known as a bronchopleural fistula.

3 Tension pneumothorax (Figure 29). The hole between the lung and the pleural space is small and acts as a one-way valve, allowing air to enter the pleural space but preventing it from escaping. The pressure in the pleural space builds up until it is above atmospheric pressure. This causes collapse of the affected lung, shift of mediastinal structures, and consequent compression of the opposite lung.

Medical and nursing problems
Chest pain or tightness
Breathlessness
— can rapidly worsen in a tension pneumothorax

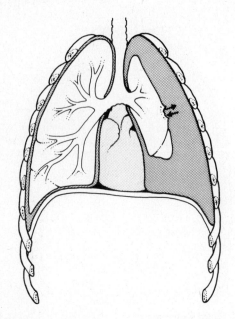

Figure 28. Open pneumothorax.

Cyanosis
— present in tension pneumothorax
— fatal respiratory failure can occur
Anxiety

Medical treatment
- If the pneumothorax is large, an intercostal drain will be inserted into the pleural space. This is then connected to an underwater seal drain (Figure 30). The 'water-seal' allows air to leave the pleural space but prevents it returning.
- Thoracic suction is sometimes necessary if re-expansion does not occur.

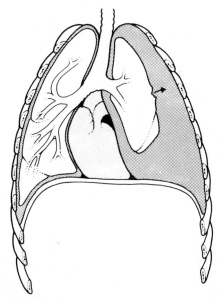

Figure 29. Tension pneumothorax.

Nursing intervention
- Pain and anxiety relief is usually instantaneous once the thoracic catheter has been introduced.
- The lower end of the tube should always be covered by the water in the drain bottle.
- The bottle should never be raised above the level of the tube insertion, or water will enter the pleural space.
- The nurse ensures that the level in the tube is 'swinging' with respiration, i.e. that it is not obstructed.
- The drainage tube should only be clamped in an emergency, for example when disconnection or breakage occurs.
- The tube is clamped when the bottle is changed. If it is accidently left clamped, a tension pneumothorax may occur because of accumulation of air in the pleural space.

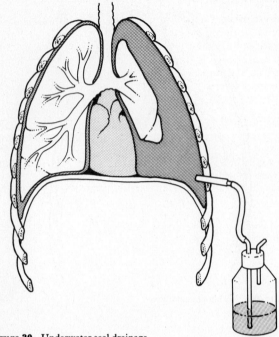

Figure 30. Underwater seal drainage.

- If blood is present in the tube, from trauma, 'milking' may be necessary using a pair of rollers, to prevent obstruction of the tube by blood clots.
- The patient can move around, providing the drain is held below waist level.
- The thoracic catheter is removed after five to six days.

Conclusion

Small pneumothoraces often resolve without intervention. Recurrent pneumothoraces can be treated surgically by performing a parietal pleurectomy (stripping of part of the parietal pleura).

Pleural effusion

A pleural effusion is a collection of fluid in the pleural space. The commonest causes are pneumonia, malignancy and tuberculosis. Transudates of fluid into the pleural space also occur in cardiac failure, renal failure, liver disease and malnutrition. The main symptom is dyspnoea.

Pleural aspiration is performed for diagnosis or treatment.

Further reading

Collins, J.V. (1979) *A Synopsis of Chest Diseases* Bristol: John Wright & Sons.

Grenville Mathers, R. (1983) *The Respiratory System* Edinburgh: Churchill Livingstone.

Nursing (1979) *Breathing* Volumes 6 and 7 (October and November).

7
Haematological Nursing

Blood is composed of:

Plasma	Cells
— 90% water	— erythrocytes
— 7% plasma proteins	— leucocytes
— inorganic salts	— platelets
— hormones	
— enzymes	
— nutrients	
— waste products	

Various nutrients are essential for the formation of erythrocytes (red blood cells). These nutrients include iron, protein, vitamins B and C, inorganic salts, and some hormones.

Clotting of blood is important to prevent severe bleeding. The mechanism of clotting is shown in Figure 31. Factors normally found in the plasma are also essential for clotting.

The following terms are used to describe abnormalities of the blood:

erythrocytosis — an increase in the number of circulating red cells

anaemia — deficiency in either quality or quantity of red cells

haemolysis — disintegration of red cells

thrombocytopenia — a decrease in the number of platelets in the blood

leucopenia — a decrease in the number of white cells, usually granulocytes, in the blood

leucocytosis — an increase in the number of white cells in the blood

Haemophilia

Haemophilia is a hereditary disorder in which the clotting power of the blood is deficient. This is due to the absence of one of the clotting factors — Factor VIII (the anti-haemophiliac globulin).

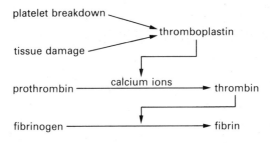

Figure 31. Mechanism of blood clotting.

This hereditary defect appears only in males, but can be transmitted by females.

Medical and nursing problems
Haemorrhage
— usually initiated by trauma
Ankylosis of joints
— deformity
— swelling
Anaemia
— depending on the extent of the bleeding

Medical investigation and treatment
● Intravenous Factor VIII or cryoprecipitate is given prior to any surgical interventions.
● Fresh blood is given to replace blood lost.
● Packs may be used to control bleeding from the nose or from a tooth socket.
● Intramuscular injections should never be given because of the risk of haematoma formation.
● When bleeding into a joint (haemarthrosis) occurs, analgesia is essential. Pethidine and other narcotic drugs are sometimes required. The incidence of addiction associated with these drugs is high.
● Deformity of the joints (ankylosis) may necessitate surgical intervention.

Nursing intervention

- If haemarthrosis occurs, the joint is rested.
- Icepacks may be useful to reduce swelling and relieve pain.
- Analgesia is given every three or four hours to relieve pain.
- Pulse and blood pressure are recorded at least four-hourly in order to detect severe blood loss.
- Patients with haemophilia are often very anxious. Careful explanation and reassurance should be given.

Conclusion

A child with haemophilia is encouraged to lead as normal a life as possible, but trauma should be avoided. Most children with haemophilia attend ordinary schools. Regular dental care is necessary to avoid dental extractions.

Genetic counselling should be given to haemophiliac men, their sisters and their daughters. Sterilization should be considered.

Anaemia

Anaemia is a deficiency in either the quality or the quantity of red blood cells, resulting in below normal levels of circulating haemoglobin.

Causes

Blood loss
— haemorrhage
— excessive menstrual loss
— chronic bleeding from haemorrhoids, peptic ulcer
Failure to produce red blood cells (aplastic or hypoplastic anaemia)
— deficiency of:
    vitamin B_{12}
    folic acid
    iron
    thyroxine
    vitamin C
— suppression of bone marrow:
    radiation
    idiopathic
    drugs
    toxins

Excessive destruction of red blood cells (haemolytic anaemia)
— abnormal red blood cells
— toxins
— drugs
— malaria
— antibodies to the rhesus factor

Medical and nursing problems
Tiredness
Breathlessness on exertion
— due to reduced oxygen supply
Pallor of the skin and mucous membranes
— due to reduced haemoglobin and blood supply to peripheries
Tachycardia
Chest pain } due to increased work load on heart
Cardiac failure
— due to decreased blood supply to cardiac muscle
Gastrointestinal symptoms
Weight loss

Iron-deficiency anaemia

This type of anaemia may be due to insufficient dietary intake of iron, to acute haemorrhage or to chronic bleeding. It is most common in women of childbearing age because of the increased iron requirements of pregnancy and lactation, and because of menstrual loss.

Medical and nursing problems
The following problems are in addition to those listed above.

Low haemaglobin
— below 10 g/100 ml (normal 13.6 – 15 g in women)
Brittle nails
Smooth, shiny, sore tongue (glossitis)
Inflammation at the corners of the mouth (angular stomatitis)

Medical investigation and treatment
● Iron preparations, e.g. ferrous sulphate, are given orally. These should be given after meals to prevent gastrointestinal

disturbances. Iron preparations are occasionally administered by intramuscular or intravenous routes.
- A blood transfusion may be necessary in severe anaemia.
- The cause of the anaemia is investigated, and treated if necessary.

Nursing intervention
- The patient is assisted to rest, especially if cardiac failure is present.
- Mouth care is given two-hourly.
- The patient is advised to eat more iron-containing food, e.g. red meat, liver, green vegetables, eggs.

Conclusion
Iron deficiency anaemia can be prevented by giving iron therapy and dietary advice to pregnant women and to those with menorrhagia.

Pernicious anaemia

This type of anaemia is caused by an inability to absorb vitamin B_{12} due to the absence of intrinsic factor in the stomach.

Medical and nursing problems
The following problems are in addition to those listed on page 117.

Sore tongue
Mouth ulcers
Lemon tint to skin   } due to the presence of bilirubin from the
Urobilinogen in urine } excessive breakdown of red blood cells
Numbness in fingers and toes
Intermittent diarrhoea
Absence of hydrochloric acid in the stomach

Medical investigation and treatment
- Bone marrow puncture will reveal large, abnormal, red blood cells.
- A Schilling test may be performed. This involves the administration of radioactive vitamin B_{12} orally and vitamin B_{12} intramuscularly. The urine is then collected for 24 hours.

- Vitamin B_{12} is given as intramuscular cyanocobalamin or hydroxocobalamin 1 mg once or twice per week initially. Thereafter a maintenance dose of 1 mg monthly is given.
- Oral iron therapy may also be given.

Nursing intervention
- The patient is assisted to rest.
- Mouth care is performed two-hourly. Mouth ulcers may be treated with a local preparation such as carbenoxolone gel.
- A well-balanced diet is given.

Care of the patient having a blood transfusion

The following complications arise during or after a blood transfusion:

pyrexia	rigors
headaches	backache
rash	vomiting and diarrhoea
jaundice	oliguria
anuria	uraemia
circulatory overload	
dyspnoea	
pulmonary oedema	
tachycardia	

Prevention of complications
A bag of blood should be checked by two nurses, one of whom should be qualified. The procedure followed involves checking:
  patient's identity
  blood group
  number of the unit of blood
  expiry date

Temperature, pulse and respiration rate are observed and recorded hourly. The blood pressure is taken prior to commencement of transfusion. A fluid intake and output chart is kept. The patient should be observed for signs of complications; the medical staff should be informed if any of the above complications occur.

Packed cells are used where there is a risk of circulatory overload. A diuretic may be given orally when whole blood is used. Drugs should not be added to blood. Dextrose is incompatible with blood and will cause coagulation if given through the same giving set.

Purpura

Purpura is a condition characterized by bleeding into the skin and mucous membranes. Haemorrhagic spots occur, the smaller ones of which are called petechiae. Purpura may occur for the following reasons:

infection, e.g. septicaemia
allergy, e.g. Henoch–Schönlein
thrombocytopenia — idiopathic or drug-induced
scurvy
defect in clotting mechanisms, e.g. haemophilia

Treatment depends on the underlying cause. In idiopathic thrombocytopenic purpura, the treatment involves the administration of blood and high doses of corticosteroids. Splenectomy is sometimes necessary.

Agranulocytosis

Agranulocytosis is a condition characterized by a marked leucopenia (too few white cells); in particular there is a great reduction in neutrophils. This condition may occur as a side-effect of drugs, e.g. cytotoxic drugs, chloramphenicol or phenyl-butazone, or radiation.

Pyrexia and sore throat occur. The white cell count is less than $2.0 \times 10^9/1$ (normal $6.0–8.0 \times 10^9/1$). The body's response to bacteria is reduced and so the patient is protected from further infection by reverse barrier nursing. Mouth care is performed at least two-hourly and the patient is encouraged to drink two-and-a-half to three litres of fluid/day. Infection with *Candida* (thrush) often occurs in the mouth, and an anti-fungal agent, e.g. amphotericin, may be prescribed. In severe cases the mortality rate is high.

Polycythaemia vera

This is a disease in which there is increased production of red blood cells. The cause is unknown.

Headache, tinnitus, dyspepsia and fatigue occur. The increased viscosity of the blood increases the risk of venous thrombosis. Treatment is with venesection, irradiation or chemotherapy.

The leukaemias

Leukaemia is a malignant condition resulting in over-production of immature white cells. The cause is unknown.

Leukaemia may be acute or chronic, and may affect any type of white blood cell.

Acute leukaemia

This condition occurs most frequently in children. The white blood cells involved are usually lymphocytic.

Medical and nursing problems

Pyrexia	Thrush *(Candida* infection)
Infections	Lethargy
Epistaxis	Breathlessness and other
Purpura	symptoms of anaemia
Bleeding gums	Joint pains
Sore throat	Irritability
Mouth ulcers	Depression

Medical treatment
- Cytotoxic drugs:
   cyclophosphamide
   vincristine
   methotrexate
   mercaptopurine
   These drugs interfere with cell division and can therefore cause unpleasant side-effects. Alopecia, vomiting, diarrhoea, and mouth ulcers may occur. Suppression of the bone marrow may result in infection and haemorrhage.
- Corticosteroids, antibiotics, antifungal agents and anti-emetics are commonly prescribed.
- Blood transfusions are used to correct anaemia.
- Nose packs may be used to halt epistaxis.

Nursing intervention
- Infection is prevented by:
    reverse barrier nursing
    mouth care at least two-hourly
    good fluid intake, i.e. 2.5–3 l/day
    meticulous personal hygiene
- Pyrexia may be reduced by fanning and by tepid sponging.
- Skin damage is prevented by changing the position of the patient at least two-hourly. Barrier cream is applied after episodes of incontinence.
- Temperature, pulse and respiration are recorded four-hourly in order to detect signs of infection and anaemia.
- Reduction of stress is important. Careful explanation is given to every patient, including children. Parents are informed of the future treatment and prognosis. Boredom should be alleviated and the aim should be to get the child home as soon as possible.
- Continuing support to the whole family is necessary.

Conclusion
Without treatment, death will occur in a few weeks. With treatment remissions occur. The survival rate for children, based on a term of 5 years, has now risen above 65%.

Chronic leukaemia

Chronic leukaemia may be either myeloid or lymphatic. It usually affects people aged 40 to 70 years.

Medical and nursing problems

Lethargy	Enlarged spleen
Breathlessness and	Epistaxis
other symptoms of	Bruising
anaemia	Enlarged lymph nodes
Abdominal pain	(lymphatic leukaemia)

Medical and nursing intervention
- Treatment involves cytotoxic drug therapy, e.g. busulphan.
- A blood transfusion may be given to correct anaemia.

● Deep X-ray treatment may be used to reduce splenic and lymph node enlargement.

Conclusion

Most patients with chronic leukaemia are able to lead a normal life. The prognosis varies from three years to a normal life expectancy.

Hospital admission is rare unless the symptoms of anaemia, infection and haemorrhage become severe.

Hodgkin's disease

This is a malignant disease of the lymphoid tissue. It is more common in men aged 20 to 40 years. The cause is unknown.

Medical and nursing problems

Enlarged lymph nodes	Pyrexia
— neck	Weight loss
— axilla	Lethargy and symptoms
— groin	of anaemia

Medical and nursing intervention
● A lymph node biopsy is performed in order to make the diagnosis.
● Cytotoxic drug therapy is given (see page 121).
● Radiotherapy may be used if the disease is localized.

Conclusion

The majority of patients live for five years or more; some are completely cured.

Further reading

Hughes-Jones, N.C. (1979) *Lecture Notes on Haematology,* 3rd edition. Oxford: Blackwell Scientific.

8
Gastroenterological Nursing 1

Disorders of the digestive system include conditions affecting the alimentary tract (Figure 32) from the mouth to the rectum. The organs associated with the alimentary tract — the liver, biliary system and pancreas — are considered in Chapter 9.

Nursing assessment of the patient with gastrointestinal disease
There are a number of problems that a nurse will consider when assessing a patient. Which problems are present will depend on the area of the alimentary tract involved. However, it must be remembered that such problems are not always caused by diseases of the digestive system.

Dysphagia — difficulty or discomfort in swallowing
Dyspepsia — indigestion
Nausea — the sensation of 'feeling sick', sometimes associated with giddiness and faintness
Vomiting — forcible ejection of the contents of the stomach
Haematemesis — vomiting of blood
Constipation — infrequent and/or difficult passage of faeces
Diarrhoea — frequent passage of loose or fluid faeces
Pain — different types of pain may be present. The nature and type of pain, e.g. retrosternal pain (heartburn), abdominal pain, pain on defaecation, is an important aid to diagnosis
Weight loss
Poor appetite
Lethargy

Investigations

Radiography
A radio-opaque substance (barium sulphate) can be used to outline the gastrointestinal tract. Which investigation is performed will depend on the area to be studied.

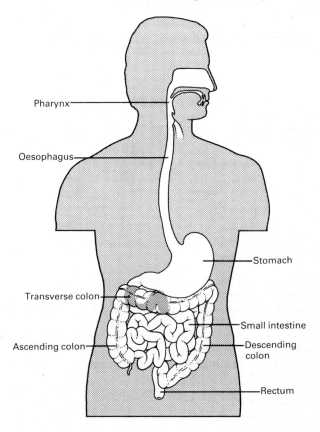

Figure 32. The gastrointestinal tract.

Barium swallow — oesophagus
Barium meal — stomach
Barium meal and follow through — stomach and small bowel
Barium enema — large bowel

Endoscopy
Endoscopes   allow   visual   examination   of   areas   of   the

gastrointestinal tract. They also can be used to take a biopsy (sample) of tissue. Which investigation is performed will depend on the area to be studied:

Oesophagoscopy — visual examination of the oesophagus

Gastroscopy — visual examination of the stomach

Colonoscopy — visual examination of the colon

Sigmoidoscopy — visual examination of the rectum and sigmoid colon

It is also possible to take biopsies of the jejunum using an endoscope.

DISORDERS OF THE MOUTH AND PHARYNX

Lesions or infections of the oral mucosa can be localized or widespread. If the mucosal involvement is widespread it is termed stomatitis; disease of the tongue is glossitis, of the lips, cheilitis, and of the gums, gingivitis.

Stomatitis

There are several types of stomatitis which vary in form from simple inflammation to vesicle formation and ulceration.

Types

1 Infection with *Candida albicans* (thrush) — a yeast-like fungus.

2 Ulcerative stomatitis — commonly seen in children who are malnourished.

3 Apthous stomatitis — a common cause of stomatitis in infants and young children. It is caused by the virus herpes simplex. Vesicles appear which may rupture and form ulcers.

Some systemic diseases such as syphilis, pernicious anaemia, leukaemia, tuberculosis, smallpox and chickenpox can cause stomatitis.

Medical investigation and treatment

- A swab or scraping from a lesion may be sent for bacteriological examination.
- Antiseptic lozenges, e.g. domiphen bromide (Bradosol), or

antifungal agents, e.g. nystatin lozenges or suspension, are given. In severe cases penicillin may be given systemically.

Nursing intervention
- Mouth care is essential and should be performed before and after eating.
- The nurse should ensure that the patient receives adequate nutrition and fluid. The soreness of the mouth and lips means that it is difficult for the patient to eat and drink without pain. A straw is sometimes helpful for taking fluids, and food may be swallowed more easily if it is soft in texture.
- Many cases are infective so care is necessary to prevent cross-infection. Disposable crockery and individual mouth care equipment is used.

Tonsillitis

Tonsillitis is an acute infection of the tonsils which involves, to varying degrees, the peritonsillar and pharyngeal tissues. The causative organism is usually *Streptococcus haemolyticus*, but a number of other micro-organisms can be responsible. It is primarily a disease of children and young adults.

Medical and nursing problems
Sore throat
Dysphagia with associated pain
Raised temperature
— may be as high as 39–40°C
Poor appetite
Malaise
Headaches may be present

Medical treatment
- Aspirin gargles, particularly before meals, or antiseptic lozenges, e.g. domiphen bromide (Bradosol) may be given to relieve soreness of the throat and mouth.
- Streptococcal infections are treated by systemic antibiotics, e.g. penicillin. This will also help to prevent the development of peritonsillar abscess (quinsy), nephritis or rheumatic fever.
- As recurrent attacks of tonsillitis can cause partial obstruction of the nasopharynx, partial deafness due to blockage of the

pharyngotympanic (eustachian) tubes, and frequent absence from school, surgery is often considered. A tonsillectomy and removal of adenoidal tissue may be performed when the patient has recoverd from the acute infection.

Nursing intervention
- Mouth care should be given two-hourly.
- The nurse should ensure that the patient receives adequate nutrition and fluid intake. Food may be swallowed more easily if soft. Hourly fluids should be encouraged.
- Bed rest may be necessary in the acute stage until the patient's temperature subsides to a normal range.

Ulceration of the pharynx

Pharyngeal ulcers have a number of causes, for example, tuberculosis or syphilitic infection, malignant growths (in particular carcinoma of the tonsillar area), or a type of sore throat known as Vincent's angina. Treatment is aimed at the primary cause.

DISORDERS OF THE OESOPHAGUS

The oesophagus is a tubular organ with a fairly simple anatomical structure and a straightforward function. Despite this, it may give rise to a complex set of symptoms from a wide variety of disorders.

Hiatus hernia

Hiatus hernia is the condition where a portion of the stomach moves up into the chest through the oesophageal hiatus (opening) of the diaphragm. In those patients who have a hiatus hernia the hernia may not be present all the time. It may occur only on lying down or when the intra-abdominal pressure rises on coughing or straining.

Hiatus hernias are usually classified into two types: (a) sliding and (b) rolling or paraoesophageal hernias.

Medical and nursing problems

Epigastric discomfort ⎫
Dyspnoea ⎬ due to slowness of hernial sac to
Palpitations ⎬ empty after meals causing mediastinal
Cough ⎭ pressure

Pain and nausea
— on beginning meals ('heartburn')
— after lying flat
— sometimes on going to bed or changing position
— on bending down for long periods, e.g. after gardening
— pain may extend down one or both arms and simulate angina

Dysphagia and vomiting
— due to oesophagitis (a sense of rawness in the gullet)

Haematemesis and anaemia
— iron deficiency anaemia with blood in the stools can occur
— massive bleeding with haematemesis can occur
— associated peptic ulceration can take place

Medical investigation and treatment
- An oesophagoscopy, barium swallow or meal and chest X-ray may be necessary to establish the diagnosis.
- The effects of oesophageal reflux are reduced by regular use of antacids, e.g. aluminium hydroxide (Aludrox), particularly after meals and before going to bed.
- Anaemia, which is normally of a simple microcytic iron-deficiency type, may require a course of iron therapy, e.g. ferrous sulphate.
- The response to medical treatment will normally be sufficient, but occasionally surgical intervention is required.

Nursing intervention
- Small bland meals should be taken, and the evening meal should be eaten at least three to four hours before retiring.
- The head of the bed should be raised by about 23 cm (9 in) to help prevent reflux into the oesophagus. Alternatively pillows under the chest or under the top of the mattress may be sufficient.
- Activities involving bending or stooping should be restricted. At home, for example, long-handled gardening tools or household equipment should be used.

- Obesity is fairly common in these patients, and the symptoms will be greatly reduced if weight reduction occurs. The patient's diet is assessed and advice given by the dietician regarding dietary restriction.

Gastro-oesophageal reflux and oesophagitis

Although reflux of acid gastric contents occurs in most people from time to time, it usually passes unnoticed. If reflux becomes frequent, symptoms may develop. Inflammation of the oesophagus — oesophagitis — can occur due to reflux of either gastric or duodenal contents. Gastric juice contains acid and the enzyme pepsin, both of which can damage the oesophageal mucosa. Duodenal contents, which contain bile and pancreatic enzymes, may reflux through the pylorus into the stomach, and in turn into the oesophagus, causing oesophagitis.

Medical and nursing problems
Pain (heartburn)
— a burning sensation in the stomach and oesophagus
— mainly retrosternal
— may radiate to back, neck, jaw and arms
— usually occurs after large meals
— exacerbated by weight gain
— precipitated by change in position e.g. bending down or lying flat
Nausea and vomiting
— due to reflux of acid contents
Pneumonia
— in severe cases
— due to aspiration

Medical and nursing intervention
- Intervention is aimed at preventing gastro-oesophageal reflux (see page 129).

Carcinoma of the oesophagus

Carcinoma of the oesophagus is primarily a disease of the elderly. Lymph node involvement occurs relatively early and there may be downward spread that can involve the liver. An oesophagoscopy with biopsies and a barium swallow will be performed to establish the diagnosis. Although carcinoma of the oesophagus has a bad prognosis, much can be done to alleviate the distress and suffering which is caused, in particular, by the accompanying dysphagia.

Medical and nursing problems
Dysphagia
— usually onset is gradual
— steadily increases in severity
Weight loss
— due to inadequate nutrition
— more marked if there is hepatic involvement

Pain is not usually present unless the disease is widespread. Despite the lack of pain, thirst and excessive salivation make this condition very distressing for the individual. Difficulty in swallowing occurs when about half the circumference of the oesophagus is involved and it may be associated with poor coordination of the oesophageal contractions. At first the patient will have difficulty swallowing solid food such as meat, but as the dysphagia increases he may become unable to swallow his own saliva.

Medical treatment
- Treatment may be either by surgery or by radiotherapy. However, as this condition is usually seen in elderly patients, they are often too ill or frail to undergo extensive surgery, and radiotherapy is usually the treatment given.
- At the present time, curative treatment has a low rate of success. Therefore palliative treatment is of correspondingly greater importance.
- When surgery is not possible, some form of intubation of the oesphagus may be performed to relieve the dysphagia. Types of prosthetic tubes used include the Souttars tube, the Mousseau-Barbin tube and the Celestin tube.
- Gastrostomy has been used to ensure adequate nutrition, but should only be used if it is thought that the patient's general health will be improved to such an extent that surgery will be possible.

Nursing intervention
- Dysphagia is uncomfortable and frightening. The patient will be anxious and distressed, and needs reassurance, full explanations and empathy.
- Thoughtful presentation of food and fluids will help alleviate distress.

Achalasia

The inability of the lower oesophageal sphincter to relax after swallowing is known as achalasia. Oesophageal motility is also abnormal. As sphincter relaxation is incomplete, the normal passage of food to the stomach is obstructed.

Medical and nursing problems
Dysphagia
— intermittent at first
Regurgitation
— common
— does not taste sour or bitter, unlike bile reflux
— worse on lying down, especially at night
Pneumonia or lung abscess
— occurs when achalasia is untreated
— due to aspiration
Chest pain
— unusual
Weight loss
— if patient reluctant to eat
— unusual

Medical treatment
Treatment of this condition is controversial. The choice lies between dilation and surgery. The majority of the patients in the United Kingdom are treated by a surgical cardiomyotomy of the Heller–Ramstedt type.

Oesophageal varices

The portal venous system communicates with the systemic venous system in the lower third of the oesophagus; here branches of the left gastric vein (portal venous system) and the oesophageal veins (systemic venous system) meet.

If the pressure in the portal venous system rises, it is transmitted from the gastric veins to the veins of the lower oesophagus and varices (dilated veins) occur. This can happen in patients with cirrhosis of the liver (see Chapter 9).

Oesophageal stricture

Chronic persistent gastro-oesophageal reflux may result in a benign oesophageal stricture. Once an established fibrous stricture has occurred it requires either surgical or endoscopic dilation. Oesophageal dilation is often performed by an endoscopic approach with the patient under light sedation (Figure 33).

Patients may require dilation at three- to six-monthly intervals. Following dilation, patients should be closely monitored for possible perforation. They may be treated with cimetidine (Tagamet) 400 mg twice daily, and an alkali after meals and before going to sleep.

DISORDERS OF THE STOMACH

Gastric and duodenal ulcers

It is common practice to describe both gastric and duodenal ulcers as peptic ulcers. However, there is considerable evidence that they have different causes, although their treatment may be similar. It is important to remember that, although duodenal ulcers are almost certainly different from gastric ulcers, they may occur together.

Some of the factors thought to be involved in the development of peptic ulcers are:

geographical location	sex
social grouping	age
occupation	blood group
diet	heredity
tobacco	hypersecretion of acid
alcohol	personality
drugs	anxiety

It is not yet possible to integrate these numerous aetiological

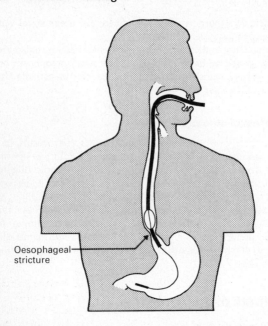

Oesophageal
stricture

Figure 33. Dilation of an oesophageal stricture using a Eder–Puestow dilator.

factors into one neat explanation, and it may be possible that peptic ulcers result from a variety of mechanisms.

Peptic ulcers may be single or multiple, large or small, acute or chronic. It is particularly important to determine whether they are benign or malignant.

Medical and nursing problems
Epigastric pain
— usually central
— may vary from over the sternum to over the umbilicus
— ranges from minimal discomfort to severe pain
— usually associated with meals
— comes on one to two hours after food
— may wake patient in early morning
— relieved by food, alkalis, vomiting

— comes in 'attacks' lasting days or weeks
Vomiting and nausea
— haematemesis
Blood in faeces
— makes faeces appear 'black'
Malaise and weakness
— due to anaemia caused by blood loss and poor nutrition
Anorexia
— due to pain caused after eating

Medical investigation and treatment
● A barium meal and gastroscopy will normally be performed to confirm the diagnosis.
● Hospital admission and bed rest are often required to help healing and avoid stress.
● Drugs will be prescribed with three aims:
    to reduce acid
    to reduce pepsin
    to increase mucosal resistance
● Antacids, e.g. Aludrox, Maalox, Gaviscon or Mucaine, buffer the acid in the stomach. They are given after meals and last thing at night. In severe cases they may be given three-hourly.
● Cimetidine (400 mg twice daily) inhibits both basal and nocturnal acid secretion, as well as acid secretion stimulated by food.
● Drugs which help inhibit pepsin and increase mucosal resistance include carbenoxolone (Duogastrone).
● Anaemia is treated by oral iron tablets, e.g. ferrous sulphate 200 mg three times daily, and/or by a blood transfusion.
● In some cases peptic ulcers cause perforation and haemorrhage and surgery will then be considered.

Nursing intervention
● Blood pressure and pulse are recorded to observe for signs of haemorrhage.
● Vomiting and fluid input and output are recorded. It is particularly important to record and report haematemesis.
● Bowel actions are recorded on a stool chart, noting whether or not blood is present in the faeces.
● Assurance and explanation is given to relieve stress or anxiety.

● Advice and education is given concerning the patient's future habits and lifestyle.

Advice on discharge

Diet/meals. In the past certain dietary restrictions were recommended, stressing the need for a bland diet with a predominance of milk-based and carbohydrate products. However, as there is no evidence that any particular diet is beneficial, patients should be advised to only avoid foods that disagree with them. This may include highly seasoned foods.

It is beneficial to take regular meals as the acidity of the stomach contents fluctuates less due to the buffering effect of food.

Alcohol. This should be stopped or reduced as it stimulates gastric acid secretion.

Smoking. Smoking should be stopped or discouraged as it hinders the healing process.

Drugs. Patients should be advised about taking drugs that may aggravate their ulcer. Such drugs include many analgesic and anti-inflammatory drugs.

Stress and anxiety. The patient will need advice, and support, on how to reduce stress in his life. It is thought that anxiety contributes to the formation of peptic ulcers and may delay healing.

This advice may be difficult for the patient to follow. It is important that the family is involved, as they can provide support and encouragement during the changes in lifestyle that may be required.

Carcinoma of the stomach

Carcinoma of the stomach is a common malignant growth. Men are affected twice as often as women; this sex ratio is fairly constant throughout the world, although the incidence of this disease varies greatly from race to race.

Gastric carcinoma is often diagnosed late and the tumour has often invaded related structures, including the lower oesophagus, pancreas and peritoneum. Lymphatic spread is common, secondary spread via the bloodstream leads to involvement of the liver, lungs, brain and bone.

Medical and nursing problems
Often asymptomatic in early stages
Anorexia ⎫
Weight loss ⎬ occur before pain
Dysphagia ⎫
Fullness after eating ⎬ develop later
Severe epigastric pain ⎭
Iron deficiency anaemia often present

Medical investigation and treatment
- The diagnosis will be made by barium meal and gastroscopy.
- Surgical resection offers the only hope of cure. Results are often poor due to the difficulty in making an early diagnosis and the subsequent likelihood of secondary involvement. Approximately two-thirds of patients have advanced disease when diagnosed and therefore only one-third are considered suitable for surgery. Of those on whom surgery is performed, few survive longer than five years.

DISORDERS OF THE SMALL AND LARGE INTESTINE

Ulcerative colitis and Crohn's disease

These two disorders are classified as chronic non-specific inflammatory bowel diseases. In both diseases the cause is unknown.

Ulcerative colitis is an inflammatory disorder which normally begins in the rectum and spreads proximally to affect a variable length of colon. It is essentially confined to the colon and does not affect the small intestine. It may present at any age, but occurs often in young adults.

Crohn's disease is a chronic granulomatosis disease of the intestinal tract. It affects all ages, although it occurs most often in young adults. The disease may affect any part of the gastrointestinal tract, but is commonly found in the colon and terminal ileum. It does occasionally present with diffuse

Table 3. Some difference between ulcerative colitis and Crohn's disease

Ulcerative colitis	Crohn's disease
Rectal bleeding and diarrhoea	Diarrhoea, often without blood
Anal lesions are not present	Anal lesions sometimes present
Extends proximally from the rectum	Disease may be patchy
Fine mucosal involvement	Submucosal involvement
Internal fistulas not present	Internal and sometimes external fistulas present
Disease may be relapsing	Disease often continuous

involvement of the stomach and the small and large intestine. It can cause strictures and fistulae. It may be associated with other diseases such as arthritis, iritis and ankylosing spondylitis.

Some of the differences between ulcerative colitis and Crohn's disease are summarized in Table 3. If only the large bowel is involved, it is particularly hard to distinguish between these two diseases.

Medical and nursing problems

Ulcerative colitis:

Diarrhoea
— blood in faeces with some mucus
— urgency of bowel action

Severe cramping abdominal pain, usually preceding bowel action

Weight loss

Weakness and lethargy

Crohn's disease:

Diarrhoea usually without blood

Recurring lower abdominal pain, may be right-sided if terminal ileum involved

Weight loss

Weakness and lethargy

Anal lesions may be present

Internal and external fistulas may be present

Medical investigation and treatment

● A barium enema, a small bowel enema, sigmoidoscopy with

biopsy, or bacteriological examination of the faeces may be performed to confirm the diagnosis.

- Medical treatment is directed towards:
  reduction of inflammation
  reduction of infection
  maintenance of nutrition
- Drugs will be prescribed with three aims:
  to reduce inflammation
  to reduce infection
  to control diarrhoea and pain
- The following anti-inflammatory drugs may be used:
  corticosteroids, e.g. prednisolone (20–40 mg daily in the acute phase)
  sulphasalazine, 2–4 g daily
  azathioprine, 100–150 mg daily

In severe cases it may be necessary to give steroids parenterally. Sometimes steroids or sulphasalazine may be given rectally in the form of suppositories or an enema.

- Antibiotics are given to reduce infection, e.g:
  metronidazole, 200–400 mg three times daily
  co-trimoxazole, two tablets twice daily
- The following drugs may be given to control diarrhoea and pain:
  codeine phosphate, 30–60 mg four times daily
  loperamide, 2–4 mg four times daily
  Isogel, 10 ml twice daily
- The nutritional status of the patient is assessed as weight loss and malnutrition are often present. Nutritional support and advice is given.
- Nutritional supplements such as iron and folic acid may be needed.
- Vitamin B_{12} may be needed if the terminal ileum is involved.
- The hydration of the patient is assessed. If the diarrhoea is severe, dehydration may be present. Intravenous fluids and potassium may then be given.
- If medical treatment alone is ineffective, surgery may be required.

Nursing intervention
- The frequency of bowel actions and the nature of the diarrhoea

is recorded. It is important to note the consistency of the faeces and whether or not they contain blood, mucus or undigested food.

- Stool specimens are obtained for culture and sensitivity, and examined for ova and parasites.

- It is helpful to have a commode near the patient's bed as they may need to defaecate urgently.

- Temperature and pulse are recorded to observe for infection, inflammation and the effectiveness of drug treatment.

- The nurse should look for side-effects of the drugs being given. The most likely are weight gain, hypertension, glycosuria and a susceptibility to infection due to steroids.

- Dietary advice and assessment are important. Appetite and food intake will be observed. The nurse can make suggestions for a change in diet or types of food if the patient has lost his appetite.

- A normal diet is usually given. Individuals are advised to leave out foods that they know exacerbate their disease. In some cases special diets or nutritional support is given.

- High-protein and high-carbohydrate diets are given if malnourishment is severe.

- A low-residue diet may be required if strictures of the bowel are present.

- Some patients find that milk and milk-based products exacerbate their diarrhoea. In these cases, a lactose-free diet may be advised.

- Most patients are young adults and tend to feel the anxiety and distress caused by the frequency and urgency of bowel actions, weight loss and general debilitation very acutely. The nurse has a vital role to play in allaying anxieties and providing support.

- It was thought that anxiety was a predisposing factor to these diseases. However, it is more likely that emotional disturbance and depression occur as a result of the symptoms.

- Explanation about treatment, an understanding of how distressing the urgency and frequency of bowel actions must be, and optimism about the future help to ease the patient's distress. Simply being aware of how a person must feel about having to go to the lavatory twenty times a day, with diarrhoea and pain on each occasion, is a help. This is a vital part of nursing people with these diseases and its importance cannot be over-stressed.

Diverticular disease

A diverticulum is a herniation of the mucosa through the muscle wall. Diverticula may occur anywhere in the gastrointestinal tract, but they are most commonly found in the colon. When diverticula become inflamed, because of faecal impaction and infection, the condition is known as diverticulitis.

The symptoms that result from the formation of diverticula vary considerably; patients are often symptom-free until a complication such as infection occurs. However, if a pharyngeal or oesophageal diverticulum occurs, its presence may cause severe mechanical symptoms.

Colonic diverticulitis is usually treated by advice on the prevention of constipation — either by dietary changes or the provision of a laxative. In severe cases, hospital admission and possibly surgery may be required.

Carcinoma of the colon and rectum

Carcinoma may occur anywhere in the large bowel but is most commonly found in the rectum and sigmoid colon.

Medical and nursing problems
The symptoms and signs will vary slightly according to the site of the tumour.

Pain
— usually not severe
— a persistant, dull ache
— sometimes associated with meals ⎱ especially in carcinoma
— patient may be afraid to eat ⎰ of the caecum
Alteration of bowel habit
— occurs most often in carcinoma of the descending colon or rectum
— alternating constipation and diarrhoea may occur
Blood and mucus in faeces
— usually means the carcinoma is low in the colon
Steady weight loss

Medical investigation and treatment
● A barium enema followed by a sigmoidoscopy or colonoscopy with biopsies will ususally confirm the diagnosis.

- Unless secondary spread has occurred, surgery will normally be performed.

Parasites

There are a wide variety of parasites which may inhabit the gastrointestinal tract. They are commonest where personal or community hygiene is poor, and in tropical or subtropical countries. A wide range of abdominal symptoms may result with general manifestations of ill health and malnutrition.

Some of the commoner parasites are:
 tapeworm
 threadworm
 hookworm
 Salmonella
 Schistosoma (Bilharzia)
 roundworm
 whipworm

Detailed information can be found in specialist textbooks.

Further reading

See page 162.

9
Gastroenterological Nursing 2

This chapter considers the medical disorders and related nursing problems of the liver, gallbladder and pancreas. The anatomical arrangement of these organs is shown in Figure 34.

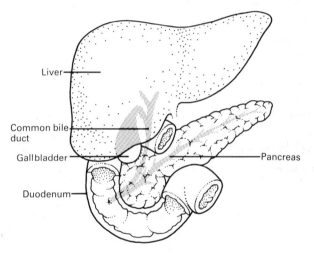

Figure 34. The liver, gallbladder and pancreas.

Jaundice

Jaundice is a term used to describe the yellow discoloration of the skin which occurs when the serum bilirubin rises above 50 μmol/1. Bilirubin undergoes a series of changes from the time it is produced in the spleen until the time it is excreted from the body. It is formed from haem following the breakdown of the red blood cell in the spleen. It is insoluble in water, and needs to be conjugated by the liver so that it can be excreted either in the faeces as stercobilinogen or in the urine as urobilinogen (Figure 35).

This pathway can be disrupted at different parts of the sequence. Table 4 shows the classification of jaundice, which depends on the part of the pathway affected.

As there are a variety of factors that can cause jaundice, it is important that an accurate history is taken from the patient concerning the sequence of his symptoms.

Table 4. Classification of jaundice

Failure to conjugate bilirubin
newborn (due to immaturity of the enzyme which conjugates
  bilirubin)
haemolytic disease
certain drugs
viral hepatitis (occasionally)
Gilbert's syndrome

Failure to excrete conjugated bilirubin
Intrahepatic
  viral hepatitis
  cirrhosis of the liver
  ulcerative colitis
  pregnancy
  carcinoma (primary or secondary)
Extrahepatic (obstructive)
  gallstones in the common bile duct
  carcinoma of the head of the pancreas
  sclerosing cholangitis

DISORDERS OF THE LIVER

Investigations

Liver biopsy

A liver biopsy is often used as an aid to diagnosis in suspected chronic disease of the liver. It is taken by puncturing the liver with a special needle inserted in the mid- or anterior axillary line between the eighth and ninth, or the ninth and tenth ribs. The

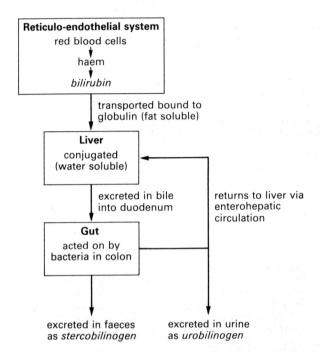

Figure 35. Bilirubin pathway.

patient's blood group, platelet count and prothrombin time ratio (blood clotting time) will have been assessed prior to this investigation. A liver biopsy is not normally performed if the prothrombin time is more than two seconds longer than the control. If the prothrombin time is raised, vitamin K may be given intramuscularly.

The equipment needed will be listed in the hospital procedure book, or see *Practical Procedures for Nurses* by H. Billing. This procedure is carried out under local anaesethesia.

Nursing intervention
- A full explanation of the procedure and of the need for supine bed rest is given to help alleviate the patient's anxiety. A doctor will obtain the patient's consent prior to the procedure.

- The patient is positioned lying supine, with his right side at the edge of the bed and his right arm behind his head so as to provide clear access to the chest wall.
- The patient may become shocked due to blood loss as the liver is an extremely vascular organ.
- The blood pressure and pulse are monitored regularly to watch for falling blood pressure and increasing pulse rate, i.e. signs of haemorrhage.
- The wound site is checked regularly for signs of bleeding.
- Bed rest in a supine position is required for 12 to 24 hours.
- The nurse regularly enquires whether the patient is in pain, as the needle may have damaged another organ.

Cirrhosis of the liver

Cirrhosis is a chronic diffuse disease of the liver, not necessarily affecting each lobule. It occurs when necrosis (death) of liver cells has been sufficiently widespread to cause the disintegration of the reticulin framework, with subsequent fibrosis and cell regeneration.

All ages may be affected, but is most common after the age of 45, when the incidence of men is twice that of women. In areas of Africa and Asia many more patients are seen in hospital with this condition than in Britain, although this pattern is changing with the rapid rise in the number of people dependent on alcohol in Western societies.

Causes

The two main causes are viral hepatitis and alcohol abuse. However, it can also develop in association with malnutrition, obstruction of the biliary tract, cardiac failure, chemical damage, and fibrocystic disease. A large number of cases have no obvious cause; the condition is then termed cryptogenic or idiopathic cirrhosis.

Clinical features

In cirrhosis of the liver, a number of main features occur:

1 *Ascites and oedema* due to low plasma albumin and portal hypertension.

2 *Portal hypertension.* The main cause is the formation of nodules by regenerating liver cells, which totally disorganize the

architecture of the liver. The mechanism for raised portal venous pressure is complex.

3 *Encephalopathy.* Liver cell damage may prevent proteins and ammonia from being broken down in the liver as normal. The result may be signs of cerebral confusion and permanent brain damage.

4 *Gastrointestinal bleeding.* Portal hypertension may cause haemorrhoids and oesophageal varices. Bleeding, particularly from oesophageal varices, is a common cause of death in cirrhosis of the liver.

5 *Jaundice.* Conjugated and unconjugated bilirubin may accumulate because bilirubin uptake and excretion are usually both defective.

Medical and nursing problems

Weakness and lethargy
Low-grade pyrexia
Jaundice
— urine dark in colour
Spider naevi
— on face, upper arms and chest
— commonly called 'spiders'
— consist of central arteriole with radiating small vessels
Memory impairment or confusion
Anorexia and weight loss
— due to gastritis
Ascites
Enlarged spleen
— due to: venous congestion
          hyperplasia of the reticuloendothelial system
Anaemia
— due to: poor appetite
          blood loss due to haemorrhoids or oesophageal varices

The patient may give a history of high and prolonged alcohol intake.

Medical investigation and treatment

- Ascites and oedema are treated by limiting dietary sodium and by diuretics, e.g. spironolactone (100 mg twice daily).

- Ascites can be treated by the drainage of ascitic fluid through a cannula. This is rarely done as it causes too great a loss of protein from the body.
- High doses of diuretics must not be used as they cause too rapid fluid loss and may cause cardiac failure.
- Portal hypertension is also treated by sodium restriction and diuretics.
- Confusion and cerebral damage will be prevented by restricting the intake of protein and by prescribing drugs to lessen protein reabsorption from the large bowel.
- The individual patient's liver function tests are assessed and his level of protein intake is determined. Theoretically, one would wish to give as much protein as possible but, due to the liver damage, a low-protein diet may be required. Protein intake in severe cases may be only 20 g daily.
- Neomycin is prescribed to prevent the breakdown of protein in the gastrointestinal tract.
- Lactulose is given to induce diarrhoea and so lessen protein absorption in the large bowel.
- Anaemia is treated by giving vitamins and iron. High alcohol intake may have limited the patient's intake of food. In particular, he will need vitamin B. Parentrovite intramuscularly and thiamine or Orovite orally will be given. Folic acid and ferrous sulphate may also be required.
- An assessment of the likelihood of gastrointestinal haemorrhage is made: the presence of haemorrhoids is noted and oesophageal varices are assessed by an oesphagoscopy or barium swallow.
- If oesophageal varices are present, a Sengstaken tube is kept by the patient's bedside in case of a sudden haemorrhage. Injection of the varices may be performed and occasionally surgical resection is considered.
- Injections of vitamin K are prescribed if the prothrombin time ratio (PTR) is raised.
- A liver biopsy may be performed.
- A chest X-ray may be necessary to detect the presence of pleural effusions which may be associated with the ascites.
- Regular blood tests are performed to monitor liver function, plasma proteins and electrolytes.

Nursing intervention
- Fluid reduction is assessed by measuring the patient's weight and girth daily, and by keeping a fluid balance chart.
- Blood pressure and pulse are observed to detect signs of bleeding.
- Bowel actions are recorded on a stool chart. In particular, the presence of blood is noted. It is vital to note whether any blood in the faeces is fresh or old (melaena). The stool chart also helps to assess the efficacy of neomycin and/or lactulose.
- Any haematemesis is immediately reported.
- The nurse should ensure a Sengstaken tube is close by the patient's bed.
- Nutritional advice and support is given to ensure the protein and sodium restrictions are followed and understood. If the appetite is poor it may be necessary to give carbohydrate supplements, e.g. Hycal.
- Observation for any drowsiness or confusion is important to ensure encephalopathy is not developing. If it does, treatment may need to be altered quickly.
- Regular temperature recordings are necessary as infection may be present or may occur.
- Chest infections are prevented by nursing the patient in an upright position and teaching deep breathing exercises.
- 24-hour urine collections are obtained to help monitor urea and electrolyte levels.
- Jaundice is monitored by testing the urine daily for bilirubin and urobilinogen.
- Psychological support is essential for both the patient and his family. Withdrawal from dependence on alcohol can be very hard, and assurance and understanding are vital.

Advice on discharge
The patient is advised to reduce, or preferably stop, alcohol consumption. General nutritional advice and guidance on the diet to be followed are given.

The nurse should ensure the importance of regular outpatient follow-up is understood. She should also try to meet the family so that support can be given concerning diet, alcohol and lifestyle alterations.

Conclusion

Cirrhosis of the liver is a debilitating disease and a high level of general nursing care will be required. Advice and psychological support is particularly important since the dietary changes and the requirement to abstain or reduce alcohol intake can put a severe strain on the patient and his family.

Viral hepatitis

More than 25% of the cardiac output at rest passes through the liver. Therefore it is particularly at risk from any organism that gains access to the general circulation or to the portal venous system.

Two viral infections of the liver are infectious hepatitis and serum hepatitis (also known as type A and type B hepatitis, respectively).

Although the presenting symptoms are similar, their epidemiology and modes of transmission differ markedly (see Table 5).

Medical and nursing problems

The history, symptoms and signs are similar for infectious and serum hepatitis. In both, a pre-icteric (prodromal) phase is followed by an icteric phase.

Pre-icteric phase:

Patient feels unwell
Nausea
Vomiting
Anorexia
Malaise
Severe headache
Loss of desire for cigarettes and alcohol
Mild fever
Urticaria
Polyarteritis (in up to 25% of patients)

Icteric phase:

Jaundice
— appears two to eight days after symptoms develop
— dark urine and pale stools

Table 5. A comparison of infectious and serum hepatitis

Infectious hepatitis (type A)	Serum hepatitis (type B)
Age Disease of children and young adults	No specific age affected
Transmission Usually via faecal–oral route, although can be through blood products	Through blood transfusions, blood products or used syringes or needles. Faecal–oral route is rare
Spread Epidemics possible as poor hygiene often an important factor. Spread may occur among members of family, within schools, closed communities, etc.	Normally sporadic spread. Constant risk for staff and patients in a haemodialysis unit
Australia antigen: Not found in the patient's serum	Usually present in serum within 12 days of onset of symptoms. May be present in the blood of healthy individuals with no symptoms; however, they are capable of transmitting hepatitis
Incubation Short period (15–40 days)	Longer period (50–160 days)

Patient begins to feel better
Appetite returns
Fever subsides
Jaundice then lessens
— stools quickly regain normal colour
— urine lightens in colour
Moderately enlarged liver
Enlarged spleen (in about 25% of patients)
Raised erythrocyte sedimentation rate (ESR)

Medical and nursing intervention
There is no specific treatment for viral hepatitis, but the following factors are important in the care of a patient with this disease.

- The patient should be nursed in a single room with full isolation precautions, e.g.
    disposable masks, gowns and gloves
    disposable crockery
    bed linen and rubbish disposed of separately
    strong disinfectant added to all urine and stools
    strict hand washing
  This should be maintained until the stools are no longer infective, which is normally seven to ten days from the onset of jaundice.
- A low-fat diet is given until the appetite returns. The diet should be high in protein and carbohydrate.
- The temperature is monitored regularly.
- Isolation precautions can cause stress. A full explanation of the reasons for these helps to ease a patient's fears.

Advice on discharge
Convalescence is important, with little exercise for three months. Alcohol is forbidden for six months to one year. Otherwise, diet may be normal. Family involvement in such advice is obviously necessary.

Advice on hygiene in the community may be required.

Conclusion
The patient is normally icteric (jaundiced) for two to six weeks. On recovery the liver returns to normal histology and function. Mortality is rare.

The failure, at present, to propagate the virus causing viral hepatitis has hampered the development of a vaccine. Human gamma globulin (750–1000 mg intramuscularly) has helped to prevent clinical hepatitis. It is of little value against serum hepatitis although work on vaccines such as hyperimmune globulin is proving of value.

Neoplastic conditions of the liver

Primary carcinoma of the liver is rare. It is normally associated with a pre-existing liver disease such as cirrhosis. However, secondary deposits in the liver (metastases) are more common. The ratio of secondary carcinoma of the liver to primary carcinoma is 20:1. Metastases usually spread from a primary carcinoma of the gastrointestinal tract, as the malignant cells are carried to the liver in the portal vein. Primary carcinomas of other organs such as the lung and the bronchus may also cause secondary liver involvement.

Treatment is normally palliative, as the primary carcinoma is usually at an advanced stage when the liver involvement is diagnosed. However, cytotoxic therapy and/or surgical resection is sometimes indicated. Liver transplantation has been achieved and there may be further developments in this field in the future.

DISORDERS OF THE GALLBLADDER AND BILIARY TREE

The common diseases of the gallbladder and extrahepatic ducts are infections (cholecystitis) and stone formation (cholelithiasis). Carcinoma is rare.

Investigations

Standard radiological techniques in investigation of known or suspected biliary tract disease include cholecystograms, percutaneous transhepatic cholangiography and ultra-sonography.

Endoscopic retrograde cholangiopancreatography (ERCP)

Endoscopic retrograde cholangiopancreatography (ERCP) has become more widely used as it enables contrast to be placed in high concentration in the biliary tree and pancreas so that excellent X-rays of the biliary and pancreatic ducts may be obtained.

It is most commonly used in investigating obstructive jaundice, disorders of the pancreas and biliary tract disease, particularly if gallstones are suspected. It is carried out under an intravenous sedative, e.g. diazepam. Certain operative techniques can be performed via the endoscope: incisions may be made electrically to allow gallstones to be passed or removed. This is especially useful in patients whose general condition may render them unfit for a laparotomy, such as the elderly.

Nursing intervention

Pre-investigation:

- The patient should have nothing orally for eight hours prior to the procedure.
- An intravenous infusion is commenced.
- Blood is cross-matched and the prothrombin time ratio checked, particularly if a sphincterotomy is to be performed.
- A full explanation is required; consent is obtained by the medical staff.

Post-investigation:

- Pulse and blood pressure are monitored to detect haemorrhage.
- The temperature is monitored to detect the presence of infection, as this investigation may cause pancreatitis. If this occurs, intravenous antibiotics will be given, e.g. amoxycillin (500 mg three times daily) and/or gentamicin (60 mg three times daily).
- The patient is usually not allowed anything by mouth for three hours following ERCP. If a sphincterotomy has been performed, the patient is not allowed anything by mouth for 24 hours.

Cholecystitis and cholelithiasis

Cholecystitis (inflammation of the gallbladder) may present as an acute, a chronic, or a subacute illness. It is more common in females and its frequency increases with age. It is usually associated with cholelithiasis (gallstones), but between 10 and 30% of those with inflammatory changes have no gallstones. Cholesterol is the major constituent of gallstones, especially in Western countries. They may be single or multiple and, in addition to cholesterol, may contain bile pigments, carbonate,

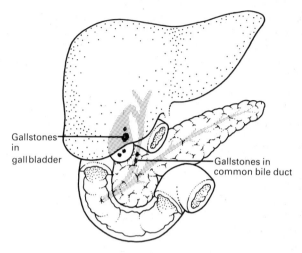

Figure 36. Gallstones.

iron, calcium, phosphate and protein. They can occur anywhere within the biliary system (Figure 36).

Causes
The aetiology of gallstones is complex and is almost certainly multifactorial.

Since cholesterol is the major constituent of gallstones, theories usually centre on cholesterol precipitation. However, there is considerable debate as to the nature of this relationship. Diet is also held to be important, and research on the effects of different types of carbohydrate is being done. Stasis, infection and alteration in the composition of bile are a further three factors thought to be relevant to the formation of gallstones. However, there is, as yet, no definitive explanation of the formation and presence of gallstones.

Medical and nursing problems
Common features on assessing the patient are:

Acute, severe pain
— deeply seated in the epigastrium
— radiates to the right hypochondrium along the phrenic nerve
— usually comes on suddenly
— reaches great intensity
Nausea and vomiting
— may be bile stained
Shock
— pallor
— tachycardia
— low blood pressure
— cold, clammy hands
Fever
— 38–39°C
Jaundice
— if bile ducts are occluded by a stone or inflammation
Tenderness and guarding of the muscles
— especially over the gallbladder

Medical treatment

- Drugs are given to relieve pain, e.g. pethidine 100 mg.
- Spasm is relieved by the prescription of an anticholinergic drug, e.g. propantheline 30 mg This lessens the spasm of the sphincter of Oddi (the valve controlling the flow of bile into the duodenum) and so decreases the pressure in the bile ducts.
- Infection will be controlled by the use of antibiotics, e.g. amoxycillin 500 mg three times daily. These may be given intravenously, or orally if the patient is able to take fluids.
- Nausea and vomiting are relieved by anti-emetics, e.g. metoclopramide 10 mg.

Nursing intervention

- Pain is assessed by regularly asking the patient. Heat pads may help with pain relief.
- The temperature is recorded regularly to detect infection and to monitor the efficacy of antibiotics. Fanning of the patient and occasionally tepid sponging may be required to lower the temperature.
- The blood pressure and pulse are monitored to detect signs of shock.

- Nausea and vomiting are relieved by aspirating the nasogastric tube hourly.
- A fluid balance chart is kept to record intravenous fluids, any vomiting, nasogastric aspiration and urinary output.
- Daily urinalysis is performed to detect the development of jaundice.
- Two-hourly mouth care is necessary as vomiting and the absence of oral fluids make a patient's mouth feel dry and sore.
- Regular washing and drying of the skin is required, as sweating and bed rest make the patient feel uncomfortable.
- Explanation and assurance are necessary as the intense pain causes a high degree of stress and anxiety.
- When the pain and fever have subsided and fluids and food are started, dietary restrictions are advised.
- Food should be low in fat content. A small amount of fat is helpful as it causes the gallbladder to contract and so prevents stasis of bile.
- If the patient is overweight, restriction of carbohydrates may be required.

Advice on discharge

The patient and his family should be seen by a dietician. Convalescence and rest may be required. This is particularly important when surgery is planned for the future.

The importance of a follow-up appointment so that future management can be planned, should be stressed.

Conclusion

Most patients with acute cholecystitis recover within a few days with conservative treatment. If gallstones are present, a cholecystectomy or ERCP and sphincterotomy may be needed. These procedures are normally performed six to ten weeks after the symptoms have subsided. In critical cases where symptoms persist, an operation may be required urgently.

DISORDERS OF THE PANCREAS

Pancreatitis and carcinoma of the pancreas are considered in this section. Diabetes mellitus will be discussed in Chapter 15.

Investigation of pancreatic disorders may include ERCP (see page 153).

Pancreatitis

Pancreatitis can take the form of an acute or chronic disease.

Causes

The cause of pancreatitis is not clearly understood and many views have been put forward. It is almost certainly multifactorial. Some factors which are thought to be important are:

Obstruction of the pancreatic ducts

Reflux from the duodenum

Infection, usually secondary; the disease develops in association with a focus of infection elsewhere in the body, e.g. viral hepatitis

Metabolic factors — hyperlipidaemia occurs frequently; also an unexplained relationship between hyperparathyroidism and pancreatitis

Vascular disorders — venous obstruction or reduced arterial supply

Alcohol

Investigations

Pancreatic function tests. Serum amylase and lipase are monitored as they reveal the degree of duct obstruction and the excretory ability of the pancreas. Pancreatic function is also assessed by taking specimens of duodenal aspirate and blood samples before and after giving injections of secretin and pancreozymin.

Radiology. An ERCP will be performed if the facilities are available. A plain X-ray of the abdomen may show pancreatic calcification.

On recovery, a cholecystogram and a barium meal are performed to look for gallbladder disease and duodenal ulcer, respectively.

Acute pancreatitis

In acute pancreatitis the changes in the pancreas vary from slight oedema to almost complete destruction by haemorrhage. Infection is not common; if it does occur it is normally secondary. Damage to the pancreas results in the escape of its enzymes both locally and into the circulation, and it is this which is reponsible for most of the patient's symptoms.

Medical and nursing problems
Epigastric pain
— usually sudden in onset
— severe and continuous
— may radiate through to the back (possibly due to the escape of blood and enzymes into the retroperitoneal space)
Shock
— rapid pulse with poor volume
— pallor
— cyanosis
— low blood pressure
Vomiting
— frequent small amounts of bile-stained fluid
— vomiting of intestinal contents occurs if peritonitis and ileus develop
Rigidity of abdominal muscles
— present, but not marked
— some upper abdominal tenderness and guarding
Fever
— if the inflammation of the pancreas is severe

Medical treatment
● Analgesia is given for the pain. Pethidine is often used as it does not cause spasm of the sphincter of Oddi. If this is ineffective morphine may be given, although this does cause spasm of the sphincter.
● The gastrointestinal tract is rested by restricting fluids and food. Intravenous fluids are given and a nasogastric tube may be inserted. Antacids, e.g. Mucaine, may be given.
● The level of sugar in the blood is monitored, as pancreatic damage can cause high blood sugar levels. If the blood sugar is high, insulin or hypoglycaemic tablets may be prescribed.
● Antibiotics may be prescribed if infection is present.
● Anti-emetics are given to relieve nausea and vomiting, e.g. metoclopramide.

- Atropine and propantheline may be prescribed to diminish vagus-stimulated secretion by the pancreas. They also help lessen spasm of the sphincter of Oddi.

Nursing intervention

- Bed rest is required.
- Local application of heat, and sometimes of cold, may be helpful in relieving pain.
- The blood pressure and pulse are recorded to detect shock. It is also necessary to observe for pallor and cyanosis.
- If a nasogastric tube has been passed, it is aspirated hourly.
- The urine is tested regularly for glucose. If glycosuria is present the nurse monitors the blood sugar using a BM Stix. This may need to be done four times daily. Urine is also tested for bilirubin and urobilinogen as obstructive jaundice can occur.
- The temperature is monitored to detect infection.
- A fluid balance chart is maintained to record intravenous fluids, vomit and urinary output. Monitoring urinary output is particularly important in pancreatitis as anuria can develop in severe cases of shock.
- Bowel actions are recorded on a stool chart, steatorrhoea may develop due to pancreatic damage.
- Mouthwashes are offered two-hourly to lessen the soreness and dryness of the mouth caused by vomiting and the restriction of oral fluids.
- Psychological support is necessary to reduce the distress caused by the severe pain.
- Dietary advice for the patient and his family may be necessary if the pancreatic damage results in high blood sugar levels.
- Alcohol is forbidden. If alcohol intake has contributed to a patient's pancreatitis, it can be difficult for him not to take alcohol again and advice and support will be necessary. Family involvement and outside support groups are essential.

Chronic pancreatitis

Chronic pancreatitis is characterized by progressive fibrosis and atrophy of the pancreas. It may occur insidiously without pain until the patient presents with obstructive jaundice, steatorrhoea or diabetes. Obstructive jaundice occurs due to the infiltration of the head of the pancreas with fibrous tissue. Although pain may not be present, if it is, as with acute pancreatitis, it is severe and intense.

Carcinoma of the pancreas

Carcinoma is found in three areas of the pancreas:
  in the ampulla
  in the head of pancreas
  in the body and tail

Carcinoma of the pancreas is rare, being about 1% of all carcinomas. Men are more commonly affected than women. Most occur in those aged 50 to 70 years, although other ages may be affected.

Medical and nursing problems
Weight loss
Pain
Indigestion
Melaena
Chronic diarrhoea
— steatorrhoea sometimes present
Mild diabetes
Venous thrombosis
Fever
Metastases in coeliac plexus of nerves
Jaundice

Medical and nursing intervention

- The location and spread of this carcinoma, together with the general condition of the patient, mean that treatment is normally palliative. The aim will be to relieve symptoms so that the patient is as comfortable as possible.
- Surgery offers the only prospect of a permanent cure. However, this is extremely difficult and in itself carries a high mortality rate. Some surgical procedures, such as cholecysto-duodenostomy, are performed to ease symptoms such as jaundice.

Further reading

Billing, H. (1981) *Practical Procedures for Nurses,* 3rd edition. London: Baillière Tindall.

Bouchier, I.A.D. (1977) *Gastroenterology,* 2nd edition. London: Baillière Tindall.

Gribble, H.E. (1977) *Gastroenterological Nursing* London: Baillière Tindall.

Hollanders, D. (1979) *Gastrointestinal Endoscopy — An Introduction for Assistants* London: Baillière Tindall.

Jones, F.A., Gummer, J.W.P. & Lennard Jones, J.E. (1968) *Clinical Gastroenterology,* 2nd edition. Oxford: Blackwell Scientific.

10
Nutrition

Nutrition is essential for human life. The basic purpose of eating is to provide the nutrients necessary to allow growth of body cells until adult stature is reached and to replenish the substances needed to maintain an adequately functioning body.

Illness has two effects on nutrition. First, the requirements for calories, protein and other essential ingredients may be altered. Second, the ability to consume, digest, or utilize these nutrients may be affected.

The role of the nurse is critical in maintaining a patient's nutrition. She is in a position to assess a person's nutritional status, advise on the dietary changes required due to a specific illness, and to help provide nutrition.

This chapter will consider the balanced diet, the assessment of a patient's nutritional needs, and the nurse's role in the provision of oral, enteral and parenteral nutrition. Dietary needs related to specific diseases are discussed in the relevant chapters.

The balanced diet

A normal balanced diet consists of:
    Proteins
    Carbohydrates
    Fats
    Mineral salts
    Vitamins
    Roughage
    Water

To function effectively, each cell in the body needs these substances. A balanced diet will contain an appropriate amount of each.

Energy requirements vary widely according to age, sex, occupation and climate. A sedentary man in hospital would need about 10 500 kJ/day, whereas a woman would need 8 800 kJ/day.

It is important to remember that in many illnesses, energy requirements and protein breakdown are increased.

Proteins

Proteins are required for growth, maintenance and repair of body tissue, for the production of enzymes, hormones, antibodies and plasma proteins, and for the production of heat and energy.

A healthy adult requires 70–100 g of protein/day. Proteins are obtained from lean meat, fish, egg whites, cheese, milk, nuts, cereals, peas and beans. Their energy yield is 17 kJ/g.

Carbohydrates

Carbohydrates are required for the production of heat and energy, for the oxidation of fats, for the formation of adipose tissue, to spare protein being used for energy production, and to provide roughage.

A healthy adult requires 400–500 g of carbohydrate/day. Carbohydrates are obtained from cereals, bread, potatoes, root vegetables, cane sugar, jam and fruits. Their energy yield is 17 kJ/g.

Fats

Fats are required for production of heat and energy, for maintenance of cell structure, to transport fat-soluble vitamins, and for the formation of adipose tissue.

A healthy adult requires 80–100 g/day. Fats are obtained from butter, cheese, cream, fat meat, oily fish, nuts, sunflower and corn oil. Their energy yield is 37 kJ/g.

Mineral salts

The most important minerals are potassium, calcium, sodium, phosphorous, iron, magnesium, chlorides and sulphur.

Potassium helps to maintain the osmotic balance between intracellular and extracellular fluid. It is essential for muscle contraction. It is found in fish, meat, vegetables and citrus fruits.

Calcium is required for the growth of bones and teeth, for the clotting of blood, and for normal muscle function. It is found in milk, cheese, flour, bread and vegetables.

Sodium is required for the formation of bone, for osmosis in the extracellular fluids, for electrolyte balance and for the flavouring of food. It is found in fish and meat. It is added to food during cooking and at the table in the form of sodium chloride.

Iron is needed for the formation of haemoglobin. It is found in red meat, liver, egg yolks, wholemeal bread and vegetables.

Phosphorous, magnesium, chlorides and sulphur are present in all foods.

Vitamins

Vitamins A, D, E and K are found in fatty food and are fat-soluble vitamins. The vitamin B complex and vitamin C are water soluble.

Vitamin A is needed for growth and for the protection of surface tissue and certain parts of the eye. It is found in animal tissues, especially in liver and liver oils. Vitamin A is added to margarine.

Vitamin D is required for the metabolism of calcium and phosphorous and therefore the growth of bone and teeth. It is found in milk, butter, fats, fish, and fish-liver oils.

The role of vitamin E in the body is unclear. It is present in all foodstuffs.

Vitamin K is essential for the formation of prothrombin in the liver. It is found in many green vegetables.

The vitamin B complex includes vitamins B_1, B_2 and B_{12}. Vitamin B_1 (thiamine) is needed for metabolism of carbohydrates. Vitamin B_2 is needed for cell metabolism. Vitamin B_{12} prevents the development of pernicious anaemia. The vitamin B complex is found in meat, liver, eggs and cereals.

Vitamin C is necessary for the formation of connective tissue and for the integrity of capillary walls. It is found in citrus fruits, root and green vegetables.

Roughage

Roughage forms the bulk of faeces and helps to stimulate peristalsis in the gastrointestinal tract. It is found in vegetables, fruits, cereals, wholemeal bread and bran.

Water

Water is present, in a high proportion, in all plants and animals.

Assessment of a patient's nutrition

There are a number of factors to be considered when assessing a patient's nutrition:

Ability to swallow and absorb food
Dietary restrictions or needs related to his illness
Physical ability to eat and drink independently
Dietary likes and dislikes
State of mouth and teeth
Cultural/religious needs or restrictions
Appetite
Number of meals normally eaten
Quantity of food normally consumed
Age and sex
Height and weight
Home environment

These factors form the basis on which the nutrition of the patient can be planned. The dietician will be involved, with the nurse, in assessing the dietary needs of the patient.

In planning an individual patient's diet, it is very important to consider his home environment. A diet given in hospital, where it can be controlled, is of limited use unless the patient understands his particular needs and is able to continue the diet when at home.

Nutrition can be given in three ways:
orally
enterally (nasogastric feeding)
parenterally (intravenous feeding)

The nurse has an important role in each of these methods of giving nutrition.

Oral nutrition

Many hospitals provide meals on a hotel-style basis. Menus are given out for the patients to complete and food is placed on individual trays, which are served and cleared away by junior nurses or non-nursing staff. Thus, the role of the nurse has been reduced. This is to the detriment of patient care, as it prevents the nurse from assessing nutritional intake and from giving advice.

Assessing nutrition at meal times

As nutrients are essential for the repair of body tissue, it is important that the nurse knows what the patients under her care have eaten. In addition, she must be aware of changes in the patients' appetites.

Knowledge of nutritional intake and appetite provides information about the health of the patient. Poor nutritional intake may indicate a deterioration in a patient's condition. Poor appetite may reflect anxiety or depression. This information is necessary to help assess medical care. Without the nurse's involvement, this knowledge is unavailable.

A further reason why nurses must be involved at meal times is that a number of patients will have dietary restrictions. They may need advice or education on what they should or should not eat. Therefore nurses must ensure that serving and clearing away food does not become a non-nursing duty.

Nursing intervention

Presentation and serving of food:
- The way food is presented and served is important in making it desirable. If food is neatly arranged on a plate, the patient will feel like eating. The principle is the same as in a restaurant, where, if food was piled up and gravy slopped over the edge of the plate, one would not want to eat it.
- Many people like a drink with their meal and this should be provided.
- If trays are used, the cutlery and condiments should be carefully arranged. Tray cloths make a surprising difference to the amount of food eaten.
- Meals should be served in a calm and unhurried manner. They are not a task to be quickly finished, but a vital part of a patient's care.

Nursing considerations:
- The nurse ensures the patient is positioned correctly. Sitting up, well supported, in a bed or chair, makes eating easier and lessens indigestion.
- The nurse ensures any aids required are present, e.g. non-stick mats, adapted cutlery, plate guards, etc.

- The nurse ensures dentures are clean and in the patient's mouth.
- Mouth care may be required before and/or after meals.
- If the food presented is not wanted, replace it with other foods or supplements of equal nutritional value.
- Food should be of the same consistency as the person is accustomed to eating at home.
- If the patient requires feeding by the nurse, this should be done in an unhurried way with the nurse sitting down. The patient should be given time to enjoy the food. It is helpful to offer fluids at regular intervals when feeding someone, as it often helps digestion. It also serves to slow down the meal and thereby counteract a tendency to complete it quickly.

Food supplements

Normal meals may not always provide adequate nutrition. Difficulty with swallowing, general malaise and debilitation, or specific dietary needs, may mean that oral food supplements are needed.

There are a variety of supplements available. Some are complete foods, e.g. Express Dairy feeds or Ensure, while others consist of specific nutrients, e.g. Caloreen or Hycal. With the help of the dietician it is possible to find a particular food supplement that the patient enjoys.

Food supplements are extremely helpful in giving the patient sufficient nutrition. He may be used to eating only one meal daily. This may not provide adequate nutrition for his particular illness or general condition. Supplements may be easier to take than an extra meal.

The early timing of the evening meal in hospital will not suit all individuals, and some may keep food in their locker. It is necessary to be aware of how much and what foods the patient is eating in this way, otherwise, the nutritional assessment is inaccurate. In addition, he may be eating food that is inadvisable, for example a patient with diabetes may be eating ordinary chocolate.

Advice on discharge

Nutrition may remain as important in maintaining health at home as it was in hospital. Dietary advice should be given on the basis of the patient's home, family, economic status, physical capabilities, (including his ability to get to the shops and cook for himself), level of understanding, particular illness and general health.

Advice should be given throughout the patient's stay in hospital. He should choose his own food, with nursing supervision, rather than be given the correct diet. This will help him learn which foods he should be eating.

The whole family should be involved, so that they understand the dietary needs required and can offer support and encouragement. This can be particularly helpful when dietary restrictions are difficult for the patient to adhere to, for example reducing diets or abstinence from alcohol.

The dietician should be involved in giving advice to both the individual and his family.

The nurse's involvement and role in oral nutrition cannot be over-stressed, as poor nutrition may delay recovery.

Enteral nutrition

Feeding via a nasogastric tube is the appropriate way of providing nutrition in any patient who cannot eat enough for their requirements *yet* have a normally functioning gastrointestinal tract.

Patients who will need nutritional support by this means are:

Patients with a low intake, e.g. anorexic or unconscious patients

Patients with disorders of the upper gastrointestinal tract, e.g. carcinoma of the oesophagus

Patients with high nutritional requirements due to catabolic states such as burns, multiple trauma or sepsis

There are two methods of enteral feeding: bolus feeding and continuous feeding.

Bolus feeding

This is becoming less common. A wide-bore tube is passed via the nose into the stomach. The prescribed feed is given every three hours using a syringe attached to the tube. The stomach contents are aspirated prior to each feed.

Bolus feeding is important when delayed gastric emptying is present. The wide-bore tube allows aspiration to be performed and

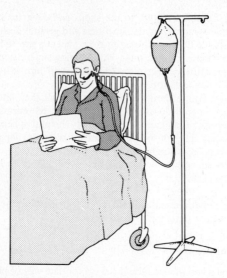

Figure 37. Continuous enteral nutrition.

thereby ensures the stomach is empty. However, this method is not often used as it is of less nutritional benefit than continuous feeding, the procedure is time consuming, and the size of the tube makes it uncomfortable for the patient.

Continuous feeding
Feeding via a fine-bore nasogastric tube is used more often than bolus feeding. A fine-bore tube is passed via the nose into the stomach. The prescribed feed is delivered continuously using a reservoir and giving set (Figure 37). Its rate of delivery is often controlled by a pump. This ensures that the feed is given at a constant rate and thereby aids absorption. These tubes are much more comfortable than wide-bore tubes. A wide variety of tubes (e.g. Clinifeed or Portex tubes), delivery systems and pumps are available.

   If the patient is being enterally fed because of a low intake or high nutritional needs, he may eat and drink in addition to the enteral feed.

Table 6. The composition of some of the commonly available enteral feeds

Feed	Packaging	Content Protein (g)	Fat (g)	Carbohydrate (g)	Na (mmol)	K (mmol)	Energy value kcal	kJ
Clinifeed 1875 ml Iso	5×375 ml	53	77	245	29	72	1875	7875
Clinifeed 1875 ml Protein Rich*	5×375 ml	150	55	350	64	108	2500	10500
Ensure 1880 ml	8×235 ml or bottle	70	70	270	61	61	1920	8064
Ensure Plus 1880 ml	8×235 ml can	103	100	375	90	92	2720	11424
Express Enteral Feed 2000 ml Standard	4×500 ml carton or 2 litre pouch	63	96	253	55	65	2064	8669
Express Enteral Feed 2000 ml High Energy	4×500 ml carton or 2 litre pouch	117	128	404	85	87	3134	13163
Fortison 2000 ml Standard	4×500 ml bottle	80	80	240	70	76	2000	8400
Fortison 2000 Energy Plus	4×500 ml bottle	100	130	358	70	76	3000	12600
Isocal 1896 ml	8×237 ml can	65	83	252	44	64	2008	8434
Nutrauxil 2000 ml	4×500 ml sachet	76	68	276	66	64	2000	8400
Triosorbon 2000 ml water + 5 sachets Triosorbon	5×85 g sachet	81	81	238	85	85	2000	8400

All figures rounded off to nearest whole number.
*The manufacturers recommend diluting each 375 ml can to 500 ml with water, giving a total volume of 2500 ml for 5 cans.

Types of feed

Patients vary widely in their daily nutritional needs and no formula is ideal for everyone. Conditions vary from starvation to the severe catabolism seen in sepsis and burns. Feeds may be made up by a diet kitchen or may come direct from the manufacturers. There are a variety of proprietary feeds available and a knowledge of their composition is necessary for prescribing enteral feeds (see Table 6). Not all of these feeds are milk based.

Nursing intervention

Bolus feeding:

- A careful explanation of the procedure should be given before the nasogastric tube is inserted.
- The position of the tube is checked by injecting air into it with a syringe, while listening with a stethoscope for the sound of air entering the stomach, or by aspirating some of the gastric contents with a syringe and testing their pH. Gastric contents should be acidic, i.e. they should have a low pH level.
- Aspiration of the gastric contents should be carried out before each feed is given.
- The temperature of the feed should be 37°C when it is given. As the feed will have been stored in a fridge, it is important to check it has reached the right temperature. Water is given after the feed to keep the tube patent, and the tube is then closed with a spigot. Fluid input and output are recorded.
- The feed must be administered slowly and by gravity. If it is given too quickly there is a danger of vomiting and aspiration of the feed.
- Drugs may be given at the same time, in liquid or powder form.

Continuous feeding:

- Explanation of the procedure is required.
- The position of the tube is checked by injecting air (see above), as it is less easy to aspirate the gastric contents. If any doubt is present, the position of fine-bore tubes can be checked by X-ray as they are radio-opaque.
- Feeds are usually given at half strength for the first 24 to 48 hours to aid absorption. They will then be changed to full strength and the volume increased so as to meet the patient's nutritional needs. Fluid input and output are recorded.

- Administration of the feed may be aided by a pump. This controls the flow so that feed is given at a regular rate.
- Fine-bore tubes should be flushed with 5 to 10 ml of water six-hourly to ensure they remain patent. However, with the consistency of modern tubes, fine-bore tubes are unlikely to block up.
- If a patient is also taking oral food and fluids, it is helpful to stop feeding via the nasogastric tube an hour before meal times, so as to encourage his appetite.
- Patients are weighed daily.
- Drugs may be given via a three-way tap.

In addition to feeding via a nasogastric tube, food is sometimes given directly into the stomach or jejunum. This is administered via a gastrostomy or jejunostomy tube.

Parenteral nutrition

Parenteral nutrition is the administration of nutrients directly into the venous circulation. It is used to promote healing and recovery and to replace lost tissue in patients when it is *impossible* to provide adequate nutrition via the gastrointestinal tract.

The types of patients who are likely to need intravenous feeding are:

Those with gross sepsis causing prolonged paralytic ileus

Those in the pre- and postoperative phases of major surgery, especially those with gastrointestinal disease

Those with severe trauma or burns

Those with severe system failure where the gastrointestinal tract needs to be rested

Many nutrient solutions are hypertonic and irritant to small peripheral veins. Parenteral nutrition is therefore usually administered into a wide central vein, where rapid dilution with blood reduces the damaging effect. Usually a catheter is inserted via the subclavian vein into the superior vena cava. The end of the catheter will remain on the anterior chest wall 8–10 cm from the clavicle (Figure 38). Sometimes the cubital, jugular, cephalic or basilic veins are used.

Electrolytes are assessed daily, and the type of feed prescribed according to the patient's particular needs. Drugs may be given with the feed.

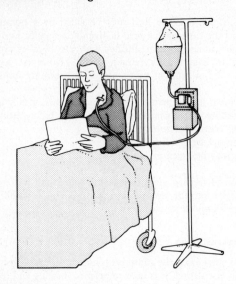

Figure 38. Parenteral nutrition.

Parenteral nutrition is a potentially hazardous therapy, as the patient is subjected to risks of:
 infection
 metabolic disturbance
 vascular damage
 emotional problems

Infection of the blood by bacteria or fungi is a potential problem because:
 Nutrient solutions are an excellent culture medium
 An inert catheter is situated in a vein for a long period of time
 The outside of the catheter provides a possible route of direct entry for organisms to the blood.

Metabolic disturbance can occur when large volumes of hypertonic solutions are infused. *Vascular damage* may occur due to:
 air embolism   catheter fracture
 catheter blockage   catheter leakage

Emotional problems may occur; being deprived of oral food and drink for a long period can cause anxiety and distress. The psychological and social needs which are normally met by eating are unfulfilled.

It is the nurse's responsibility to minimize these risks and to ensure the parenteral nutrition is administered safely.

Nursing intervention

Infection control:
- Asepsis must be carefully maintained during all procedures concerned with parenteral nutrition. Changing the infusion set and performing the dressing to the catheter where it emerges onto the skin are the two main procedures performed.
- The inclusion of all the nutrient solutions needed, including the fat emulsion, in a single container has reduced the risk of infection, because the infusion set needs to be changed only once every 24 hours.
- Individual hospitals have their own procedures for changing infusions, which should be based on the British Intravenous Therapy Association's guidelines.
- The nurse records the patient's temperature six-hourly, and observes the skin at the catheter entry site to look for signs of infection.

Metabolic disturbance:
- Accurate control of the infusion rate is essential because sudden or slow infusion of nutrients such as glucose or potassium causes severe metabolic disturbance. There are a variety of mechanical devices available, perhaps the most beneficial of which is the volumetric pump.
- The urine is tested for sugar six-hourly. It may be necessary to also directly measure blood sugar. Glycosuria may suddenly appear if the feed has been administered too rapidly.
- A careful record of fluid input and output is kept. This should be done from parenteral feed to parenteral feed and not from 12 midnight to 12 midnight. It may be necessary to collect urine or other fluid over 24 hours to estimate nitrogen and electrolyte loss.
- The patient is weighed daily. Any signs of oedema are reported.

Vascular damage:
- The nurse should take great care with the equipment used.
- Using Luer-lock connections, securing the tubing by adhesive tape, using an extension tube between the catheter and infusion set, and using atraumatic clamps when the intravenous set is disconnected will all help prevent vascular damage.

Emotional problems:
- The nurse can help allay some of the feelings of anxiety and distress by having a positive attitude. Parenteral nutrition is not permament; it is a form of treatment needed only until the main problem is resolved.
- Exercise is important, where practical, for both psychological and physiological reasons. It provides a change of environment and helps assure the patient that he is recovering.
- Mouth care helps in both an emotional and physical way. Sucking of boiled sweets can be particularly beneficial.

Parenteral nutrition is life-saving for many patients. It is an important method of nutritional support, and its use is increasing. The nurse must remember that, even with good organization, parenteral nutrition remains a potentially hazardous therapy.

Further reading

Beck, M.E. (1980) *Nutrition and Dietetics for Nurses,* 6th edition. Edinburgh: Churchill Livingstone.

Huskisson, J.M. (1980) *Nutrition and Dietetics in Health and Disease* London: Baillière Tindall.

Ministry of Agriculture, Fisheries and Food, Great Britain (1982) *Manual of Nutrition,* revised edition. London: H.M.S.O.

Nursing 2 (1982) *Nutrition* Volumes 4 and 5 (August and September).

11
Renal and Urological Nursing

The urinary system (Figure 39) is concerned with:
 Excretion of the end-products of protein metabolism
 Regulation of electrolyte and water content
 Regulation of acid-base balance
 Excretion of drugs and poisons
 Regulation of blood pressure
 Formation of red blood cells

The functional unit of the kidney is the nephron (Figure 40). The glomerulus filters blood so that water, electrolytes, glucose, amino acids and waste products flow down the nephron. In the tubule most of the water is reabsorbed together with the glucose, amino acids and some salts. Anti-diuretic hormone regulates the reabsorption of water.

Approximately 1.5 l of urine passes out of the tubules each day. This is conveyed from the pelvis of the kidney down the ureters to the bladder and urethra.

The following terms are used to describe abnormal function of the urinary tract:
 Retention — inability to pass urine from the bladder
 Retention with overflow — urine is voided but there is a residue of urine left in the bladder
 Anuria — failure of the kidneys to excrete urine
 Oliguria — reduction in the amount of urine excreted
 Polyuria — increase in the amount of urine excreted
 Haematuria — presence of blood in the urine
 Glycosuria — presence of glucose in the urine
 Proteinuria — presence of protein in the urine

Investigations

Examination of the urine
1   *Volume.* Normal range is 600 to 2000 ml per day.

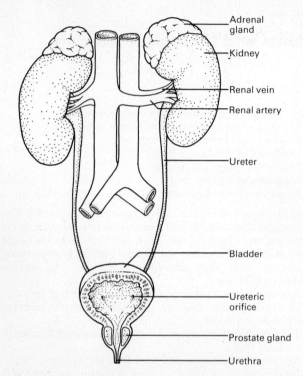

Figure 39. The male urinary tract.

2 *Specific gravity.* Normal range is 1003 to 1030. A low specific gravity indicates concentrated urine.

3 *pH.* Urine is usually acid pH 4 to 6, but becomes alkaline if left to stand. Urinary pH can be measured using a Multistix.

4 *Colour.* Dilute urine is a pale, straw colour. Concentrated urine is a darker yellow. Red or smoky-coloured urine may contain blood. Yellowish-brown urine may contain bile.

5 *Abnormal constituents.* Blood, glucose, ketones, protein, bilirubin and urobilinogen can be detected by testing with a Multistix.

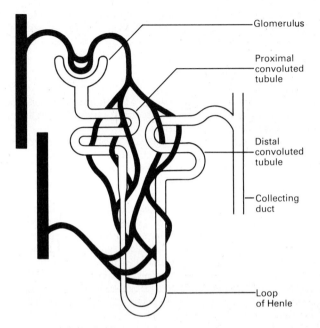

Figure 40. The nephron.

Bacteriological examination of the urine
A mid-stream specimen of urine should be obtained for microscopy and culture.

To detect the presence of tuberculosis of the urinary tract, all of the first urine specimen of the morning needs to be be sent to the laboratory.

Blood urea and electrolytes
These tests are used to detect impaired renal function. Impaired excretion of urine due to diseased kidneys will cause the blood urea and potassium to rise.

Creatinine clearance
The function of the kidneys can be measured by the clearance of

creatinine. Creatinine is an end-product of muscle function. It is filtered off in the glomeruli. Calculation of the serum creatinine, the urinary creatinine and the urine volume in a 24-hour period can be used to measure the glomerular filtration rate.

X-rays of the urinary tract

A plain X-ray of the abdomen will show the outlines of the kidneys and the presence of any stones in the urinary tract. Small kidneys may indicate chronic renal failure.

An intravenous urogram (pyelogram) involves an intravenous injection of a contrast medium which is subsequently excreted by the kidneys and therefore the outlines the pelvis and calyces of the kidney, the ureters and the bladder. It will reveal any abnormality in shape or size and any obstruction or deformity. A laxative is normally given the day before the examination in order to prevent the urinary tract being obscured by a constipated, gas-filled bowel. Better pictures are obtained if the urine is concentrated and the patient should be deprived of fluid before the test (this may be contraindicated in renal failure and myeloma).

A retrograde pyelogram involves an injection of contrast medium into the kidneys via ureteric catheters inserted through a cystoscope. The dye outlines the pelvis and calyces of the kidney and the ureter.

A renal arteriogram involves an injection of contrast medium into the aorta close to the renal arteries. To do this a catheter is passed up into the aorta through a femoral artery in the groin. The renal blood supply can then be outlined. This investigation is often performed under general anaesthesia. Vital signs and distal pulses are recorded because of the risk of haemorrhage from the arterial puncture site. The patient should rest in bed for 8 to 24 hours.

Isotope scanning of the kidney

A radioactive isotope is injected intravenously. This is taken up by the tubules of the kidney and a sensor device enables a picture of the isotope concentration in the kidney to be built up.

Ultrasound

Ultrasound of the kidney can detect structural abnormalities such as polycystic kidneys (see page 197).

Renal biopsy
A renal biopsy involves the obtaining of a minute cylinder of kidney tissue for histological examination. This is usually performed using a needle. It is a potentially dangerous procedure for which signed consent is required. Blood is cross-matched in case haemorrhage occurs. The procedure should be explained carefully to the patient. It is performed under local anaesthesia. The patient should rest in bed for 24 hours after the procedure. Observations are initially made every 15 minutes. All urine is tested for blood.

Cystitis

Cystitis is defined as inflammation of the bladder.

Causes
Cystitis is most commonly due to bacterial infection. It is more common in women because of the short urethra. Sexual intercourse often predisposes to cystitis by causing trauma to the urethra. Pregnancy and childbirth distort the anatomy of the urinary tract resulting in stasis, which also predisposes to cystitis.

The organism commonly involved is *E. coli*, which usually enters the bladder through the urethra.

Medical and nursing problems
Frequency of micturition
Dysuria
— pain and burning sensation on passing urine
Strangury
— an intense desire to pass more urine although the bladder is empty
Urine abnormal
— strong smell
— cloudy

Medical investigation and treatment
● A mid-stream specimen of urine is obtained for bacterial examination.
● Antibiotic therapy is commenced. Co-trimoxozole (Septrin) is

the most commonly used anti-bacterial drug for *E. coli* infections.

Nursing intervention
- The patient is encouraged to drink at least two-and-a-half litres of fluid each day to reduce the symptoms of dysuria and to discourage multiplication of the infecting organisms.

Conclusion
The symptoms usually disappear within 48 hours of commencement of antibiotic therapy.

Recurrent urinary tract infections should be investigated as an abnormality of the urinary tract may be present.

Women who are prone to cystitis after sexual intercourse should be advised to empty their bladders before going to sleep.

Acute pyelonephritis

Acute pyelonephritis is an acute bacterial infection of the renal pelvis and kidney substance.

Causes
Acute pyelonephritis is usually due to ascending infection from the bladder. *E. coli* is the organism most commonly involved. Other organisms which may cause acute pyelonephritis include *Klebsiella*, *Proteus*, *Enterobacter* and *Pseudomonas*.

Pyelonephritis is far more common in women than in men.

Medical and nursing problems
Pain   Dysuria
— loin pain and tenderness   Frequency of micturition
Fever   Urine abnormal
— 39–40°C   — strong smell
— rigors   — haematuria
Malaise
Confusion in the elderly

Medical investigation and treatment
- A mid-stream specimen of urine is obtained for bacteriological examination.
- Antibiotic therapy is commenced.
- Analgesics, such as paracetamol and buprenorphine, are used to relieve the loin pain. Intramuscular pethidine (50–100 mg) is given for more severe pain.

Nursing intervention
- The patient is encouraged to drink two-and-a-half to three litres of fluid each day in order to reduce the urinary symptoms and to prevent dehydration due to the fever.
- The patient is fanned or sponged if the temperature rises above 39°C.
- Temperature, pulse and blood pressure are recorded six-hourly. A rise in blood pressure may indicate deteriorating renal function.
- A fluid input and output chart is kept in order to detect a reduction in urine output.

Conclusion
In recurrent acute pyelonephritis a daily dose of antibiotics may be given long-term. An intravenous urogram (pyelogram) is performed in order to detect any abnormality of the renal tract such as renal stones. In the absence of any abnormality, recurrent acute pyelonephritis rarely results in chronic renal failure.

Glomerulonephritis

Glomerulonephritis is an inflammatory non-bacterial disease of the glomeruli. There are three types:
   minimal change
   proliferative
   membranous

In each of these types, protein leaks through the glomeruli and appears in the urine.

Causes

Glomerulonephritis is caused by an immunological or allergic reaction affecting the glomeruli.

A common antigen causing acute proliferative glomerulo-nephritis is the bacteria β-haemolytic streptococcus. This organism causes a throat or skin infection, and 10 to 14 days later an allergic inflammation occurs in the kidneys. However, in many cases, the antigen causing glomerulonephritis is unknown.

Medical and nursing problems

Oedema
— generalized
— most noticeable in the face
— due to salt and water retention
Oliguria
Haematuria
Proteinuria
Hypertension
Dyspnoea
— due to pulmonary oedema
Fever
Uraemia
— raised blood urea and creatinine

Medical investigation and treatment

- Fluids are restricted to 500 ml each day plus the previous day's output.
- Dietary protein is also restricted, if necessary, to 20–40 g/day. Sodium and potassium intake may also be limited.
- Diuretic and antihypertensive drugs may be required.
- If a throat or skin infection is present, swabs will be taken and an antibiotic prescribed, e.g. penicillin.
- Blood will be taken for urea and electrolytes. A 24-hour urine collection may be necessary to estimate the creatinine clearance.
- After a period of two to three weeks, the urinary output increases, proteinuria decreases and the blood pressure returns to normal. During this diuretic phase fluid intake is increased to prevent the patient becoming dehydrated. Dietary restrictions are lifted and salt supplements may be given.

Nursing intervention
- The patient is encouraged to rest in bed.
- Mouth care should be offered two-hourly as the oral intake will be restricted.
- The patient should be weighed daily in order to detect fluid gain or loss.
- An accurate fluid intake and output chart is essential.
- Temperature, pulse, respirations and blood pressure are recorded six-hourly.
- Careful explanations about fluid and dietary restrictions are given.

Conclusion
The majority of children suffering from acute glomerulonephritis will recover completely. In adults the disease will often progress, eventually leading to chronic renal failure.

Nephrotic syndrome

Nephrotic syndrome is not a disease but a collection of symptoms. It is characterized by oedema, proteinuria and a low serum albumin.

Causes
Glomerulonephritis
Amyloidosis
Diabetic nephropathy

The excessive loss of protein in the urine results in a low serum albumin. This in turn causes a low osmotic pressure in the blood and consequently generalized oedema occurs.

Medical and nursing problems
Proteinuria
— large amount on Multistix testing
— dark foamy urine
Oedema
— puffy eyes in the morning
— swollen feet and ankles later
— oedematous genitalia

— peritoneal and pleural effusions
Mild hypertension
— due to salt retention
Susceptibility to infections
Premature artheroma
— due to hyperlipidaemia

Medical investigation and treatment

- The amount of protein lost in the urine is estimated from a 24-hour urine collection.
- A high-protein, low-salt diet is given. A low-fat diet may be prescribed if there is hyperlipidaemia.
- Diuretic and antihypertensive drugs are given.
- Nephrotic syndrome caused by glomerulonephritis can be treated with steroids, e.g. prednisolone. If the symptoms fail to resolve, cyclophosphamide, an immunosuppressive and cytotoxic drug, may be used.

Nursing intervention

- Urine is tested daily for protein and blood.
- The patient is weighed daily in order to detect fluid gain or loss.
- An accurate fluid intake and output chart is kept.
- Temperature, pulse and respirations are recorded six-hourly.
- Blood pressure should be recorded with the patient lying and standing as postural hypotension may sometimes occur. The patient may find anti-embolic stockings helpful.
- Unnecessary pressure on the oedematous areas should be avoided as pressure sores develop readily. Strict cleanliness is essential to avoid infection.

Conclusion

The course of the disease is variable. The patient often has multiple hospital admissions and is very conscious of his oedematous appearance. He will need continuing support and explanation.

Many patients will develop chronic renal failure, except for those suffering from minimal change glomerulonephritis.

Acute renal failure

Acute renal failure is severe but temporary renal damage causing a uraemic state. The condition is potentially reversible.

Causes
Impaired blood supply to the kidneys
— severe haemorrhage
— extensive burns
— dehydration
— shock
— severe infections
— myocardial infarction
— crush injuries
— poisons
    chemicals
    drugs
— incompatible blood transfusion
— major surgery
Renal causes
— acute glomerulonephritis
— fulminating pyelonephritis
Obstruction to outflow of urine
— prostatic hypertrophy
— renal stones
— tumours
— strictures

Medical and nursing problems
Oliguria, anuria
Proteinuria
Haematuria
Shortness of breath
— pulmonary oedema
— heart failure
Uraemia
— nausea, vomiting, diarrhoea
— confusion and twitching
— hyperventilation
— pruritis

Hypertension or hypotension
— due to sodium excess or deficiency
High serum potassium
— may cause cardiac arrhythmias
— cardiac arrest may occur (any level above 6 mEq/l is
dangerous)

Medical investigation and treatment

- Fluid intake is restricted to 500 ml each day plus the previous day's output.
- A mid-stream specimen of urine is taken for bacteriological examination and specimens from other sites may be required.
- Antibiotic therapy is commenced if infection is present.
- Dialysis is usually required as a matter of urgency if pulmonary oedema is a problem.
- Protein intake is restricted to 20–60 g/day depending on the severity of the renal failure. Sodium intake is restricted to 20–40 mEq/day (20–40 mmoles/day) and potassium to 20–40 mEq/day (20–40 mmoles/day).
- Anti-emetic drugs, e.g. metoclopramide, may be required before meals to prevent nausea and vomiting.
- Kaolin mixture, diphenoxylate (Lomotil) or loperamide are used to relieve diarrhoea.
- Chlorpheniramine (Piriton) is used to relieve pruritis.
- Hypertension can be controlled with drugs such as hydralazine, atenolol and minoxidil.
- Hypotension due to sodium deficiency may be corrected with a sodium chloride infusion or with slow sodium tablets.
- If the serum potassium is above 6 mEq/l (6 mmoles/l) cardiac arrhythmias may occur. An ion exchange resin (Calcium Resonium) is given orally or rectally to reduce the potassium level.
- If Calcium Resonium is ineffective, glucose and insulin are given intravenously to promote the transfer of potassium ions into the cells, thus lowering the serum potassium. An infusion of sodium bicarbonate may also be helpful.
- Peritoneal dialysis or haemodialysis, if necessary, are used early on in the illness. Dialysis is the most effective method of reducing the urea and creatinine levels and of controlling the serum potassium. Dialysis is discussed on page 191.

- Fits may occur in severe uraemia and the patient may require an anticonvulsant drug, e.g. phenytoin.
- Blood is taken frequently to measure urea and electrolytes levels. Blood cultures are taken if the patient develops a fever.
- The diuretic phase of acute renal failure occurs 10 to 21 days after the onset. Increasing amounts of urine are passed; these are very dilute at first. Renal function gradually improves, although it may be several months before it returns to normal.
- During the diuretic phase, fluid and electrolyte balance must be watched carefully. Fluid intake is calculated as before. Sodium and potassium supplements may be required and the dietary restrictions may be lifted.
- Urine collections for creatinine clearance will be performed in order to assess renal function.

Nursing intervention
- The patient with acute renal failure is very seriously ill and will be very dependent on the nursing staff. Careful explanation to the patient and his family is necessary at all times.
- The patient is weighed daily in order to assess fluid gain or loss. An accurate fluid intake and output chart is kept.
- Temperature, pulse, respirations and blood pressure are recorded at least six-hourly. Fever is often present as these patients are very susceptible to infections. Blood pressure is measured lying and standing.
- Urine is tested daily for blood and protein.
- If the patient is short of breath he should be assisted to sit upright and the medical staff should be informed. Oxygen is given as prescribed.
- In more severe pulmonary oedema, it is helpful if the patient sits in a high-backed chair with his legs down. This allows excess fluid to pool in his legs rather than in his lungs.
- Sputum in pulmonary oedema will be frothy and possibly blood-stained.
- The protein- and electrolyte-restricted diet should be high in calories to prevent the breakdown of tissue protein. Glucose solutions such as Hycal and Caloreen are used to increase calorie intake.
- Frequent mouthwashes, or ice to suck, are necessary as the patient may feel thirsty and may have an unpleasant taste in his mouth.

- Patients with acute renal failure are lethargic due to uraemia and anaemia. Care is needed to relieve pressure on the skin and so prevent skin breakdown.
- Strict attention is given to personal hygiene as these patients are susceptible to many infections.
- Careful washing and drying of the skin is essential after episodes of incontinence. A barrier cream such as zinc and castor oil should be applied to the buttocks.

Conclusion
The prognosis for a patient with acute renal failure varies according to the original cause. The prognosis is worse in patients who are over the age of 50, in those who have prolonged oliguria, and in those with infections. A minority of patients are left with permanent renal failure.

Chronic renal failure

Chronic renal failure is irreversible impairment of renal function.

Causes
The main causes of chronic renal failure are:
   glomerulonephritis
   pyelonephritis
   polycystic kidneys (see page 197)
   malignant hypertension

Other less common causes include diabetes, analgesic misuse, tuberculosis and amyloidosis.
   Glomerulonephritis often accompanies collagen diseases such as systemic lupus erythematosus (SLE), polyarteritis nodosa (PAN) and scleroderma.

Medical and nursing problems
Chronic renal failure will cause disturbance of most systems of the body.

Skin
— pallor due to anaemia
— scratch marks due to pruritus

Urinary
— oliguria, anuria
— proteinuria

— bruising due to platelet deficiency

Gastrointestinal
— nausea and vomiting
— diarrhoea
— anorexia
— thirst
— hiccoughs
— dry, coated tongue

Cardiovascular and respiratory
— hypertension
— chest pain
— oedema
— dyspnoea
— frothy sputum
— hyperventilation

Blood
— anaemia
— lethargy
— bleeding tendency

— haematuria

Neurological
— insomnia
— lack of concentration
— drowsiness
— confusion
— coma
— fits and twitching
— numbness in legs

Muscular
— cramps
— weakness

Bone
— pain
— osteomalacia

Eyes
— deteriorating vision

Endocrine
— impotence
— menstrual disturbances

Medical and nursing intervention

The management of chronic renal failure includes dietary restrictions, fluid and electrolyte adjustment, and, if indicated, dialysis and transplantation. The complications of renal failure are also treated. Dietary, fluid and electrolyte control are discussed on page 188.

Patients with end-stage renal failure who cannot be treated with dialysis or transplantation will require terminal care.

In the early stages of chronic renal failure most patients have polyuria and therefore the fluid intake should be liberal. In the later stages the urine output decreases and the patient will then have to restrict his intake to 500 ml each day plus the previous day's output.

When the patient can no longer be kept alive using conservative measures, dialysis may need to be considered. There are two types of dialysis — peritoneal dialysis and haemodialysis.

Dialysis is the transfer of solutes across a semi-permeable membrane from a solution of high concentration, the blood, to one of low concentration, the dialysate. Water and small molecules, such as urea and potassium, are able to pass through the membrane. The dialysis fluid is constantly removed and replaced with fresh fluid.

Peritoneal dialysis. In peritoneal dialysis the peritoneum is used as the semi-permeable membrane. The peritoneum is a large area richly supplied with capillary blood.

A cannula is inserted into the peritoneal cavity. This can be a semi-rigid cannula inserted under local anaesthesia, or a flexible Tenckhoff catheter (Figure 41), which is usually inserted under general anaesthesia. The patient is usually catheterized prior to insertion to reduce the risk of bladder perforation.

A peritoneal dialysis giving set is connected to the cannula (Figure 42) and one to two litres of warm dialysis fluid are run into the peritoneal cavity and left there for a specified period, e.g. 20 minutes. It is then run out into a sterile collection bag. This procedure is repeated until the patient's condition is stable, usually for several days. The peritoneal dialysis is then performed intermittently, as directed by the medical staff.

The three common types of peritoneal dialysis solution are 1.36%, 3.86% and 6.36% dextrose. The higher the concentration of dextrose, the more fluid is removed from the patient.

Prevention of peritonitis is essential and a strict aseptic procedure is followed when changing the bags of dialysis fluid and emptying the effluent bag.

The patient should be weighed daily (with an empty peritoneal cavity). Blood pressure is recorded six-hourly.

Continuous ambulatory peritoneal dialysis (CAPD) is a system of peritoneal dialysis which can be performed by the patient at his own home or work (Figure 43). Three to five exchanges of dialysis are performed each day. The success of this method depends on the patient's scrupulous attention to cleanliness.

Automated peritoneal dialysis machines are increasingly being used in hospitals with a consequent reduction in infection rate. They can also be used in the patient's home.

Haemodialysis. In haemodialysis an artificial membrane such as cuprophane is used. Blood is passed between layers of cuprophane and then returned to the circulation. The other side of the membrane is bathed in dialysis fluid and the waste substances diffuse from the blood into the dialysis fluid. The blood between

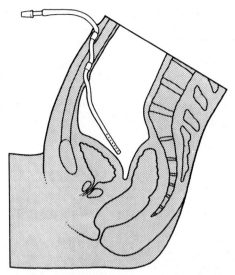

Figure 41. A Tenckhoff catheter in position.

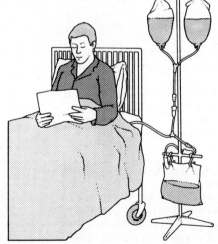

Figure 42. Peritoneal dialysis.

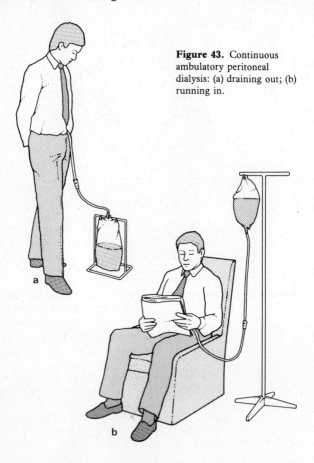

Figure 43. Continuous ambulatory peritoneal dialysis: (a) draining out; (b) running in.

the layers of cuprophane is prevented from clotting by the addition of heparin.

The patient and his family may be trained to perform haemodialysis at home. The patient is weighed before and after dialysis and the blood pressure is recorded hourly.

In order to perform regular haemodialysis, access to the circulation must be available.

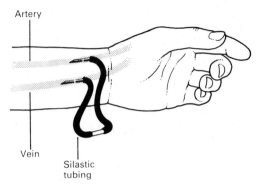

Figure 44. A Scribner shunt.

A *Scribner shunt* (Figure 44) is a loop of silastic tubing connecting an artery and vein. When required for dialysis the shunt is clamped and taken apart at the middle connection. The arterial end is then connected to the arterial tubing of the kidney machine, and the venous end to the venous tubing.

A *Cimino fistula* (Figure 45) is a subcutaneous anastomosis between an artery and a vein, usually in the arm. The vein becomes dilated, enabling needles to be introduced into the arterialized vein. These needles can be connected to the tubing of the kidney machine.

Transplantation. Renal transplantation from a live or cadaver donor is an alternative to dialysis in end-stage renal failure and gives the patient a chance to live a more normal life. Steroid and immunosuppressive drugs are used to combat rejection.

Survival rates are between 70–80% at one year compared with 90% or more after one year on dialysis.

Selection of patients for dialysis and transplantation. Both peritoneal and haemodialysis are now used in the long-term treatment of chronic renal failure. Peritoneal dialysis is the simpler method and is often the treatment of choice when dialysis is required urgently.

Selection of patients for dialysis and transplantation is dependent on a number of factors:

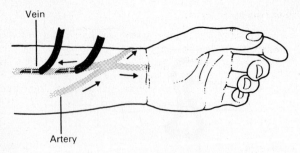

Figure 45. A Cimino fistula.

1 *Age.* The very young and the very old do not do well on haemodialysis. Peritoneal dialysis is proving increasingly useful for these people.
2 *Marital status.* Married adults are more likely to be selected for haemodialysis (as a partner is required to assist with home haemodialysis).
3 *Intelligence and personality.* The patient must have the ability to learn and cooperate.
4 The presence of other associated diseases makes dialysis and transplantation difficult.

Terminal care. If a patient with end-stage renal failure is not suitable for dialysis or transplantation there will come a time when conservative methods of treatment fail.

It is of utmost importance to relieve the unpleasant symptoms of uraemia such as vomiting and chest pain. An anti-emetic drug, e.g. prochlorperazine, can be given in conjunction with diamorphine. Oral fluids are given as required as the patient is usually very thirsty and has an unpleasant taste in his mouth. Mouth care should be performed at least two-hourly and the patient's position should be changed frequently.

The relatives should be kept completely informed and encouraged to help with the patient's care.

Death often occurs suddenly as a result of the high serum potassium causing cardiac arrest.

Polycystic kidneys

This is a hereditary progressive cystic condition of both kidneys causing chronic renal failure in middle age. The kidneys become very large with multiple cysts. It causes episodes of haematuria and loin pain. The patient will eventually require dialysis or transplantation. Bilateral nephrectomy is sometimes indicated because of chronic infection in the cysts.

Renal calculi

Stones may form in the renal tract. These stones are usually formed of calcium salts. Predisposing factors are:

Excessive loss of water by sweating

Urinary tract infection or stasis

Increased excretion of calcium, e.g. in metabolic disorders, prolonged bed rest, excess of calcium in the diet

Renal colic occurs when the stone enters the ureter. The conservative treatment of renal colic is to give the patient three litres of fluid in 24 hours. The urine is sieved and any stones found are sent for biochemical assay.

Analgesia, e.g. pethidine, is required. If the patient fails to pass the stone, surgical intervention will be necessary.

Hypernephroma

Hypernephroma is the most common carcinoma affecting the kidney. The patient presents with pain in the loin and haematuria. Metastatic deposits occur, especially in the lungs. Nephrectomy is necessary and this is followed by deep X-ray or cytotoxic therapy.

Tuberculosis of the kidney

Tuberculosis of the kidney is always secondary to a primary infection in the lungs. The patient presents with frequency, dysuria and loin pain. Early morning urine specimens are cultured for acid-fast bacilli (tubercle bacilli). Antituberculous therapy is commenced (see page 99).

Further reading

Gabriel, R. (1980) *A Patient's Guide to Dialysis and Transplantation* Lancaster: MTP.

Gabriel, R. (1981) *Renal Medicine*, 2nd edition. London: Baillière Tindall.

Scott, T., Deane, R.F. & Callander, R. (1982) *Urology Illustrated* Edinburgh: Churchill Livingstone.

Uldall, R. (1983) *Renal Nursing*, 3rd edition. Oxford: Blackwell Scientific.

12
Rheumatological Nursing

The rheumatic diseases are among the commonest of all diseases. They represent one of the most important causes of physical suffering and economic loss from illness in any nation. Diseases affecting the bones and joints are characterized by local pain, often of a persistent and chronic nature, and by varying degrees of limitation of movement and deformities. Consequently they are crippling diseases which have serious implications for the individual, his family and the community.

Rheumatoid arthritis

Rheumatoid arthritis is a common and very crippling inflammatory disease of the joints. It is a peripheral symmetrical inflammatory disease of synovium leading to destruction of cartilage and adjacent bone, resulting in deformity and loss of function of any of the 187 synovial joints in the body. The erosions can be seen radiologically.

Although at least half a million people in Great Britain alone suffer from this painful and crippling disease, the cause is not fully understood. No single initiating factor has been isolated, although it is thought that immune overactivity plays an important role. Females are more commonly affected than males in a ratio of 3:1. Rheumatoid arthritis occurs world wide and all age groups are affected, although the maximum incidence of onset is in the fifth decade.

Diagnosis is based on clinical examination and a history of the illness. Investigations which will help confirm the diagnosis are X-rays, screening of the blood for rheumatoid factor, erythrocyte sedimentation rate (ESR), white blood cell count, alkaline phosphatase levels, uric acid levels, and haemaglobin levels, in addition to other usual haematological tests. Occasionally fluid from an inflamed joint will be examined.

In cases of severe immobility, a replacement of a joint may be considered. Hip and knee joints are the joints most commonly replaced, but ankle and shoulder joint replacements have been performed.

Medical and nursing problems

These will vary considerably due to the extent of the disease and the particular joints involved. The onset may be insidious, with pain in one or two of the smaller joints, such as those of the fingers and toes, which then progresses and involves the wrist, elbow, shoulder, hip and knee joints. The changes lead to ankylosis (fixation of the joints) with a loss of movement (Figure 46). Deformity is made worse by wasting of the muscles.

In an acute phase problems include:
   Morning stiffness
   Tenderness or pain on movement for a period of days or weeks
   History of swelling of the joints
   Subcutaneous nodules may be present
   Weight loss
   Loss of appetite
   Malaise
   Raised temperature

Care of a patient with rheumatoid arthritis

In the absence of a cure for rheumatoid disease the treatment and management must be aimed at controlling the inflammatory response and preventing further structural damage.

A team approach is required, involving physicians, physiotherapists, social workers and the nurse in full consultation with the patient and his family.

The pace at which patients move about and care for themselves is often slow. Ward routine needs to be adapted to this pace so that every encouragement is given to initiative and self-sufficiency.

Care can be divided into three stages:
   rest phase
   remobilization
   rehabilitation

Rest phase

General care:
- Bed rest is required due to general malaise, and the heat, swelling and redness of the joints.

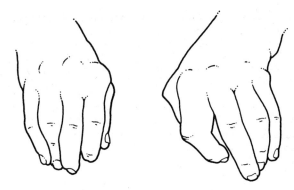

Figure 46. The hands of a patient with rheumatoid arthritis.

- The bed should have a firm mattress; fracture boards may be required.
- Pillows are positioned to ensure maximum comfort.
- A bed cradle may be used to prevent the pressure of bed clothes on painful joints.
- Changing a patient's position every two hours is important to prevent the skin becoming sore and red.
- Pressure sores can develop as bed rest, difficulty with independent movement, the firm mattress, perspiration if the patient is febrile, the presence of subcutaneous nodules on bony prominences, and malnourishment all put the skin at risk.
- Elimination of faeces and urine may be difficult, and a commode or raised lavatory seat may be easier to use than a bedpan or urinal. A high roughage diet and aperients will help prevent constipation.
- Help will be necessary with hygiene as bed rest, difficulty with movement, pain and perspiration make independence difficult.
- Support and encouragement are important as distress, depressive feelings and anxiety are felt at the loss of independence and the pain.
- If a patient is malnourished, a high-protein and high-calorie diet may be required.

- If a patient is obese, a reducing diet will be required to reduce the stress and pressure on the weight-bearing joints.
- Assistance with feeding may be necessary if the joints of the hands or arms are involved. Feeding aids such as adapted cutlery, non-stick mats, beakers, plate guards or straws can be provided (Figure 47).

Alleviation of pain:

- Pain relief forms a major part of the treatment for rheumatoid arthritis. All patients should be given regular analgesia.
- Many drugs are used to relieve the type of pain characteristic of rheumatoid arthritis. One of the commonest is acetylsalicylic acid (aspirin). This can be provided in soluble or enteric-coated form. It may be given in doses of up to 4 g/day in an acute phase. As it is a gastric irritant, it should be given with food or a glass of milk.
- There are also a wide variety of drugs which have combined analgesic/anti-inflammatory effect. Such drugs include indomethacin, phenylbutazone, ibuprofen and naproxen.
- Corticosteroids, e.g. prednisolone, may be required if the inflammation is severe.
- There are many other drugs that are used, such as gold or penicillamine, and it is vital that the nurse and patient are aware of their side-effects so that complications can be noted and avoided.
- Pain may also be relieved by resting splints, aspiration of effusions and by local injections into the joint. Heat pads or ice packs are sometimes beneficial.

Prevention of deformity:

- Correct positioning in bed will prevent further joint deformity.
- Splints (Figure 48) may be required when the joints affected are not being used, e.g. at night. These help to prevent flexion deformity and are particularly useful for knee, wrist, elbow and finger joints. They will also help to alleviate pain. The occupational therapist and the physiotherapist will help in assessing joint deformity and making the correct splint.

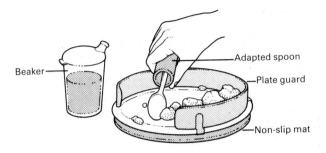

Figure 47. Feeding aids.

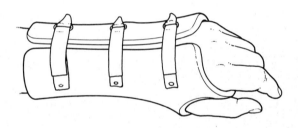

Figure 48. A resting splint.

Nursing observations:
- Temperature is recorded, as the patient may be febrile.
- The condition of the skin is observed as pressure sores may develop.
- Urinalysis and blood pressure may be recorded to detect the side-effects of certain drugs, e.g. corticosteroids may cause hypertension and glycosuria, penicillamine may cause proteinuria.
- The effectivenss of analgesia is monitored.
- The general morale and attitudes of the patient are observed.

Remobilization

- The role of the physiotherapist will be very important in planning a programme of remobilization.
- It usually begins with general exercises designed to regain muscle tone and progresses to exercises to increase muscle strength and the mobility of the joints. These exercises will be developed over a period of time. Hydrotherapy may aid remobilization.
- The nurse has an important role in supervising the exercises and ensuring that the programme is followed correctly.

Rehabilitation

- During this last phase, patients are independent within the limitations of their disease.
- They should be encouraged to wear their own clothes and go to the day room for meals.
- The nurse ensures the patient knows how to do his own exercises and how to use any splints that may be required, and knows which drugs he is to take and their side-effects.
- The social worker is often involved to ensure any problems at home or work are eased as far as is possible.

In addition to the direct care a nurse will perform, she has a vital role as a coordinator of the many disciplines involved in the care of patients with rheumatoid arthritis.

Osteoarthrosis

Osteoarthrosis is a disease in which pathological wear in the joints occurs. Advancing age is accompanied by degenerative changes affecting all the tissues of the body to a varying extent. Osteoarthrosis or degenerative joint disease represents the degenerative process affecting the joints. The term osteoarthrosis is preferred to the old term of osteoarthritis, as the latter term implies that there is an inflammatory basis for the condition. Osteoarthrosis is a very common form of joint disease, particularly in the elderly.

There are two types of osteoarthrosis — primary and secondary. Primary osteoarthrosis involves many joints and is idiopathic, i.e.

the cause is unknown. Secondary osteoarthrosis frequently involves only one joint and there is an obvious predisposing cause, e.g. a previous fracture.

Medical and nursing problems
Pain in affected joint(s)
— two types of pain
    venous (constant deep ache)
    ligamentous (sharp pain on weight bearing)
Progressive loss of movement in joint
Swelling and redness of joint

Medical and nursing intervention
In contrast to rheumatoid arthritis, this is a disease of the joints alone rather than a general disease. The pain is not caused by inflammation, therefore pain relief is often given by drugs which are only analgesics rather than those which are also anti-inflammatory drugs.

Physiotherapy is often helpful in alleviating pain in the joint and, more particularly, for strengthening the joint and increasing the degree of mobility. Hydrotherapy is sometimes beneficial as the warmth of the water helps relax the muscle spasm and the buoyancy reduces the weight borne by the joint, so allowing greater movement.

Diet is only important if the patient is obese, as this will put unnecessary strain on weight-bearing joints. In such cases an appropriate reducing diet will be started.

In cases where immobility is severe, surgery will be considered.

Infections

Some people experience arthralgia (aching in the joints) or myalgia (aching in the muscles) during the course of an infection. Occasionally musculoskeletal symptoms form part of an infectious disease and, rarely, the joint itself may be the site of an infection.

Infection within a joint is a very serious condition as it can destroy the joint and may be life threatening. Pyogenic organisms, tuberculosis and brucella can cause infection of the joints. Diagnosis is made by aspirating fluid from the joint for microbiological examination. Once an organism has been isolated, an appropriate antibiotic will be prescribed. Most antibiotics can be given systemically as they penetrate into the synovial fluid, but occasionally local administration of an antibiotic will be required.

Some infections give rise to a reactive synovitis, although infection is not present in the joint. Such diseases include brucellosis, Reiter's disease, syphilis and gonorrhoea.

Viral infections
Aching of joints and muscles is usually due to a virus infection, and the aching subsides with the fever. Viral infections such as rubella (German measles) or mumps may cause synovitis.

Gout

Gout is caused by an accumulation of excess amounts of uric acid in the body. Uric acid is produced mainly from breakdown of nucleic acids which are found in the nuclei of cells. Some uric acid is therefore normally found in the blood and urine. High levels of uric acid in the blood may be due to one of the following mechanisms: there may be an over-production of uric acid; there may be under-excretion of uric acid by the kidney; or there may be a combination of these two. Surgery has been known to provoke an acute attack of gout.

Medical and nursing problems
Pain in the affected joint
— commonly the metatarsophalangeal joint of the big toe
— sudden onset
— excruciating pain
— redness and swelling
Temperature may be raised
Nausea and vomiting may be present

Medical and nursing intervention
The treatment of gout is aimed at relieving the severe pain. The traditional drug used was colchicine but this has largely been superseded by indomethacin and phenylbutazone. However, a drug which is now being used widely is allopurinol. This

interferes with the formation of uric acid by inhibiting the enzyme xanthine oxidase.

When a patient is in bed it is essential to use a bed cradle, as even the pressure of light bed clothes on the affected joints causes excruciating pain. In hot weather it is important to ensure that the patient has a high fluid intake to prevent the formation of urate crystals in the kidney.

Diet is not now thought to be of major importance in the treatment of gout, although patients are advised to moderate their alcohol intake and to refrain from having high purine foods such as liver, kidneys, peas and beans.

Ankylosing spondylitis

Ankylosing spondylitis is a progressive inflammatory disease affecting predominantly young males. It is characterized by spinal rigidity and limitation of chest expansion. Its cause is unknown. Unlike rheumatoid arthritis, it affects both the synovial and cartilagenous joints.

Medical and nursing problems
Pain and stiffness in lower part of back
— unrelieved by rest
— worse in the morning
Chest pain
— due to involvement of costo-vertebral joints (where ribs join spine)
Rigidity of chest movement
— chest expansion is limited
— breathing is usually diaphragmatic (causing abdominal bulging or ballooning)
Anorexia
Loss of weight
Synovitis
Iritis
Postural changes
— lumbar spine flattened
— upper thoracic spine bent
— neck craned forward
— chest flattened
— known as 'Bechterer stoop' or 'hang dog' appearance
— fusion of spine can result causing a rigid 'poker back'

Medical treatment

- Analgesia is prescribed during the active phase; the drug most commonly used is soluble aspirin.
- Anti-inflammatory drugs such as phenylbutazone, indomethacin and naproxen are also given.
- Corticosteroids are not usually given, but may be necessary if the disease is progressing or if the eyes are threatened by severe iritis.
- Radiotherapy and surgery were considered in the past, but are now rarely used.

Nursing intervention

- Mobilization is vital. Patients are encouraged to exercise in order to prevent postural abnormality and limitation of movement of the spine, chest and peripheral joints.
- Exercises are taught initially by the physiotherapist and continued by the patient at home.
- Hydrotherapy is beneficial and swimming should be encouraged.
- The patient should lie on a firm bed with a supportive mattress or, if appropriate, fracture boards under the mattress.

Rheumatic fever

Rheumatic fever or acute rheumatism is mainly a disease of children and young adults. It is associated with haemolytic streptococcal infections. However, it is not direct infection by these organisms which causes the disease, but a probable abnormality in the body's immune response to the invading streptococci. The streptococci may have originally caused a mild infection, such as a sore throat, and then, due to the possible abnormality of the immune system's response, go on to cause acute rheumatic fever and rheumatic heart disease. Improvement in social conditions and the use of penicillin has meant that the incidence of this disease is declining.

The main features of this disease are polyarthritis, chorea and carditis, of which carditis is the most important as it may cause permanent damage to the heart.

Medical and nursing problems
Fever
— usually 38 – 39°C
— may be higher
Joint pains
— many joints involved for short periods
— pain moves from joint to joint
— joints are hot, red, tender and swollen
Subcutaneous nodules
— vary in size
— may be large swellings
— may be barely palpable
Skin rash
— on trunk and limbs
Malaise
Lethargy
Anorexia
Weakness
Cardiac damage
Chorea
— involuntary muscular spasm
— usually involves face and hands
— emotional lability
— also known as St Vitus' dance

Medical investigation and treatment
- Bed rest is needed to lessen the risk of cardiac damage. Periods of up to six weeks used to be required but this length of time is now rarely needed.
- An electrocardiograph (ECG) will be performed to determine whether cardiac damage is present.
- Drugs are prescribed to reduce fever, control infection and ease pain.
- Aspirin (1 – 2 g four-hourly) is given to relieve pain and bring the temperature down. Large doses may cause toxic symptoms such as nausea, headache, deafness and ringing in the ears. If these occur, the dosage is reduced.
- Penicillin may be prescribed. It does not directly affect the inflammation in the joints but combats the infection, e.g. the tonsillitis, which may have been the precipitating cause.

- Corticosteroids, e.g. prednisolone, may be prescribed if cardiac involvement is suspected. This is to lessen the risk of the heart valves becoming thickened and deformed. The development of surgical techniques have greatly improved the prognosis of patients with rheumatic heart disease. However, heart valve involvement remains the main cause of disability and death in rheumatic fever.
- Joint deformity is prevented by physiotherapy and the application of light splints.

Nursing intervention

- Temperature is recorded hourly in the acute stages to monitor the fever and the effectiveness of aspirin. Fanning and tepid sponging can be used to help reduce the temperature.
- A high fluid intake is maintained to lower the temperature and to prevent dehydration which may be caused by profuse sweating.
- Washing of the skin and a change of nightwear is required after sweating attacks to aid the patient's comfort.
- Light splints, positioning of pillows and a bed cradle are used to support joints, prevent deformity and ease pain.
- Blood pressure and pulse are recorded regularly to assess the general condition of the patient.

Diffuse connective tissue disease

This group of diseases, formerly called collagen diseases, may affect the connective tissue throughout the body. Their effects are widespread, and the involvement of many different systems of the body means they are encountered in both medicine and surgery. In addition to the two diseases described, there are three other main diffuse connective tissue diseases: systemic sclerosis, polymyositis and dermatomyositis.

Systemic lupus erythematosus (SLE)

This is a diffuse disorder of connective tissue associated with vasculitis. It has a variety of manifestations. It commonly presents with arthralgia, fever, malaise and weight loss. A rash often occurs on the face. Pleural and pericardial effusions are frequent, and atelectasis (collapse) may occur at the lung bases.

Involvement of the kidneys occurs in about one third of patients. In addition, central nervous system involvement is being recognized more frequently. The cause is unknown.

Diagnosis of this disease may be difficult. It is based on the clinical picture and a series of haematological investigations.

Treatment consists mainly of drug therapy. Corticosteroids are the main drugs used. Analgesic and anti-inflammatory drugs may be given for the joint pain. Avoidance of sunlight and the use of corticosteroid cream may help the facial skin rash.

Unless there is involvement of the renal system, the prognosis is improving steadily as treatment becomes more effective.

Polyarteritis nodosa (PAN)

This disease involves the inflammation of the medium-sized and small arteries and is characterized by segmental vessel wall necrosis. Arteries throughout the body may be involved. The cause is unknown. Polyarteritis nodosa occurs more commonly in males than females and, although it may start at any age, it is most common in young adults.

The features of the illness are widespread. A patient will present with malaise, weakness, pyrexia and weight loss. Peripheral neuropathy, heart failure, alterations in gastrointestinal function, joint pain and kidney involvement may occur. This latter problem may lead to hypertension and renal failure. Diagnosis is made by examination of a biopsy of the affected part; muscle or kidney biopsies are commonly used.

Treatment is normally with high-dose corticosteroids; doses of 60 mg/day may be given.

Further reading

Elliott, M. (1979) *Nursing Rheumatic Disease* Edinburgh: Churchill Livingstone.

Panayi, G.S. (1980) *Essential Rheumatology for Nurses and Therapists* London: Baillière Tindall.

Swinson, O.R. & Swinburn, W.R. (1980) *Rheumatology* London: Hodder & Stoughton.

Wright, V. & Haslock, I. (1977) *Rheumatism* London: William Heinemann Medical.

13
Dermatological Nursing

The structure of the skin is shown in Figure 49. The skin has the following functions:

Protection
— keeps bacteria out of the deeper tissues
— seals in tissue fluids
— waterproofs
Manufacture of vitamin D
— by the action of sunlight
Regulation of body temperature
— sweating
— vasodilation
— vasoconstriction
Secretion of oil
— waterproofs the skin
Sensation
— heat
— cold
— touch
— pain

The following terms are used to describe skin lesions:

Bullae — large blisters
Ecchymoses — large purple blotches due to extravasation of blood; do not disappear on pressure
Erythema — redness of the skin
Excoriation — removal of an area of the epidermis, leaving a red, raw surface which exudes serum
Fissures — cracks in the epidermis
Keratosis — thickening of the horny layer
Lichen — a collection of papules
Macules — a discoloration of small areas with no alteration in surface level
Papules — small, solid, raised spots
Petechiae — small haemorrhagic spots

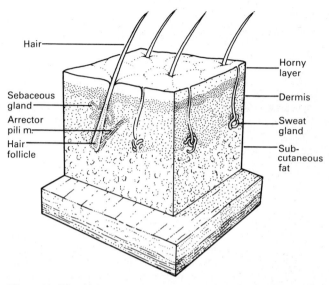

Figure 49. The skin.

Plaques — patches of the skin, harder than normal and usually raised above the skin surface

Pustules — small swellings containing pus

Vesicles — small blisters

Weals — localized oedema in the dermis

Nursing a patient with a skin disorder

Medical and nursing problems

Skin lesions

— bleeding

— scaling

Itching

Body odour

Risk of infection

Psychological problems
— self-consciousness
— social isolation
Immobility
— difficulty walking
— difficulty using hands
Loss of fluid
— exudate
— bullae

Nursing intervention
- The patient with a skin problem needs a lot of emotional and practical support. He may be very self-conscious about the unsightliness of his skin lesions and any associated odour or discharge.
- The doctor will often prescribe topical treatment for the skin lesions. The nurse should follow the instructions carefully. Types of treatment which may be used are discussed below.
- *Baths* are used to remove exudate or crusts. Medicated baths may be prescribed, e.g. potassium permanganate.
- *Lotions* are used to cool the skin and to relieve itching, e.g. calamine lotion.
- *Paste,* a thick topical application is applied using a gloved hand or a wooden spatula. Tubular gauze is placed over the paste. It is removed using arachis oil.
- *Ointments* are greasy applications which may be rubbed in. Tubular gauze is used to cover the area.
- *Cream* is a cooling application. Creams need to be reapplied three to four times daily.
- *Paints* are applied to the affected area using cottonwool or a paint brush.
- *Occlusive dressings* may be used. Polythene is used to seal off a treated area for 12 to 48 hours. Paste-impregnated bandages may be used and are left in place for two to three weeks.
- Itching may be very troublesome in skin disorders. The patient is encouraged to rest and mild sedation may be indicated. Excessive heat is avoided and light cotton clothing is worn. Itching may particularly be a problem at night. Food and drink which may cause flushing should be avoided, e.g. spices or alcohol.

- Body odour may be reduced by bathing and frequent changes of clothing. Pure soap and emulsifying ointment are suitable cleansers. The skin should be patted dry using a soft towel to avoid damaging the skin. Potassium permanganate baths may be prescribed to reduce the risk of secondary infection.

Dermatitis

Dermatitis is inflammation of the epidermis.

Contact dermatitis

Contact dermatitis is the result of an acquired sensitivity to substances which reach the skin from outside the body. These substances may be irritants or allergens. Acute contact dermatitis follows a single exposure to the substance responsible whereas chronic contact dermatitis occurs after multiple exposures.

The pattern of the eruption may indicate the cause. For example, face powder, cream, rouge and lipstick produce dermatitis limited to the face and dermatitis due to dusts and vapours may affect the eyelids.

Medical and nursing problems
Red swollen vesicular eruptions
Itching
Weeping
Scaling

Medical investigation and treatment
- Identification and removal of the cause is essential.
- Patch testing involves the application of a small portion of the suspected substance to an area of the skin not involved by the dermatitis. Several patch tests may be performed using different substances. The tests are left in position for 48 hours. A positive reaction consists of an area of inflammation beneath the suspected material.
- In mild cases a bland cream such as aqueous cream may be applied to the affected area. If the lesions are on the hands, cotton gloves should be worn for dry work and PVC gloves for wet work.

- In severe cases, corticosteroid creams may be used as sparingly as possible. They should not be used on the face.
- Secondary infection is treated with systemic antibiotics.
- Antihistamine drugs are used to control itching, e.g. promethazine hydrochloride (Phenergan).
- Sedatives may be necessary at night, e.g. nitrazepam, temazepam.
- Widespread dermatitis may occasionally be treated with systemic corticosteroids, e.g. prednisolone (10 mg three times daily).
- In chronic dermatitis the skin may become thick and scaly. Zinc and salicylic acid (Lassar's paste) may be applied to the skin in these cases.

Nursing intervention
- Dressings should be used to separate all skin surfaces.
- Limbs should be covered with tube gauze.
- Bed rest may be necessary in order to reduce oedema of the affected limbs.
- Careful explanation is necessary in order that the patient can avoid contact with the substances responsible for the dermatitis. In some cases he may need to consider changing jobs.
- The patient is advised to avoid detergents and to use soap sparingly.

Atopic eczema

Eczema is an itching, vesicular skin eruption for which there is no apparent external cause. *Atopic eczema* is a genetically determined disorder closely associated with allergic rhinitis (hay fever) and asthma. A family history is present in 70% of patients. Eczema may start in babies around the age of three months. The condition gradually improves but may relapse in adolescence.

Medical and nursing problems
Redness and scaling
— starts on scalp and face
— spreads to limbs and nappy area
Dry, itchy skin

Secondary infection
Sleeplessness

Medical treatment

- Mild sedation may be necessary at night. Diphenhydramine hydrochloride (Benadryl) or promethazine hydrochloride (Phenergan) are suitable.
- Bland preparations, e.g. emulsifying ointment, aqueous cream or E45 cream, may be used to combat dryness. Bath oil may also be helpful.
- Steroid creams may be used on active areas, but the face and flexures should be avoided.
- If infection is widespread, systemic antibiotics are indicated.
- Coal tar occlusive bandages covered with gauze may be used on the limbs. These are left in place for a week at a time.
- Vaccination should be avoided when the eczema is active.

Nursing intervention

- The family as a whole needs great support. The parents may be over-anxious and the child insecure and self-conscious.
- Careful explanation and reassurance is given.
- The child should lead as normal a life as possible.
- Most children with atopic eczema eat a normal diet, but occasionally a particular food, e.g. fish, may produce an urticarial reaction and should be avoided.

Impetigo

Impetigo is an infection of skin caused by the micro-organism *Staphylococcus*. It is common in children. *Staphylococcus* may be transferred from the nose to the skin by the hands and introduced into the skin by scratching.

Impetigo appears on exposed areas of the face, hands and knees. Vesicles form and are followed by crusting. Fresh lesions appear and spread daily.

Local treatment is with a neomycin–bacitracin ointment or with chlortetracycline (Aureomycin). Secondary infection may occur, when systemic antibiotics may be indicated.

Acne vulgaris

Acne vulgaris commences at puberty. It results from over-activity of the sebaceous glands. The hair follicle becomes blocked with keratin and micro-organisms cause an inflammatory reaction. Red papules occur and these may form pustules and cysts. Comedones (blackheads) are also present. The most commonly affected areas are the face, neck, back, chest and upper arms. Acne may persist into the mid-twenties.

Local treatment involves the use of detergents, such as cetrimide, to de-grease the skin. Sulphur applications are useful. Retinoic acid (Retin-A) loosens the keratin plug in the hair follicles and helps to eradicate comedones. Ultraviolet light and systemic antibiotics may also be used.

Erysipelas

Erysipelas is a streptococcal infection of the skin, usually of the face. The organisms enter through a break in the skin, and inflammation, oedema and blistering occur, spreading over the face. The eyes are closed due to oedema of the eyelids. The patient has a pyrexia of 39°C or more and rigors may occur. Treatment is with penicillin.

Herpes simplex

Herpes simplex is a common viral disease. Sixty per cent of people are infected and remain carriers for the rest of their lives. The virus remains dormant, erupting occasionally, especially in association with the common cold. Small ulcers appear in the mouth and vesicles appear on the face and neck. Necrotic crusts form after rupture of the vesicles. The infection subsides in about ten days.

Idoxuridine (IDU) solution may occasionally be used to treat recurrent lesions of the skin.

Herpes zoster (shingles)

Herpes zoster is a painful rash caused by the chickenpox (varicella) virus. It is generally believed that herpes zoster is due to reactivation of the chickenpox virus which has lain dormant in a sensory nerve root ganglion of the spinal cord since a primary infection with chickenpox years before. Herpes zoster may also occur three to seven days after exposure to varicella.

The virus attacks a posterior root ganglion of the spinal cord and travels along a sensory nerve fibre to reach the nerve endings. A rash occurs in a continuous line or in patches in the area supplied by the nerve affected. Vesicles are produced which eventually form necrotic crusts. Very severe pain occurs with the eruptions.

The ophthalmic branch of the trigeminal nerve is involved in 10 to 15% of patients. In such cases, corneal ulceration may occur.

Treatment is with idoxuridine (IDU) painted onto the affected area two-hourly, or with cytarabine injections for three successive days. Local antibiotic cream helps to prevent secondary infection. Pain can be relieved with analgesic drugs. In herpes affecting the ophthalmic nerve, the eye can be treated with atropine 1% eye drops and antibiotic ointment.

Herpes zoster is infectious in the vesicular phase; contacts tend to develop chickenpox rather than shingles.

Neuralgic pain may continue following an attack of shingles.

Fungal infections

Common fungal infections are caused by *Candida albicans,* tinea pedis (athlete's foot), and other forms of ringworm.

Candidiasis (thrush)

Infection with *Candida albicans* (thrush) can be present in the mouth, on the skin or in the genital region.

In adults, thrush may occur in the mouth after treatment with antibiotics or steroids, or in debilitated patients. White spots occur on the tongue and the buccal mucosa. Treatment is with nystatin suspension (100 000 units six-hourly) or with amphotericin lozenges.

In infants, oral infection may be followed by infection with *Candida* in the nappy area, axillae and neck. Treatment is with nystatin cream.

Candida skin infection is often seen in diabetic adults. Commonly infected areas include the groins, axillae and the submammary area. *Candida* balanitis may occur in the male and *Candida* vaginitis in the female. Treatment of the skin lesions is with nystatin ointment or clotrimazole (Canestan) cream. Good control of the diabetes will help to prevent these infections.

Tinea pedis (athlete's foot)
Tinea pedis is a type of ringworm. It is a common infection, particularly amongst those who share bathing facilities. Scaling and fissuring occur between the toes, and secondary infection may follow. Treatment is with griseofulvin (500 mg daily) for six to eight weeks. Local fungicidal applications are also available.

Other forms of ringworm
Ringworm appears as ringed lesions on any part of the skin or scalp. Treatment is with griseofulvin as above.

Skin infestations

The most common skin infestations are scabies and lice.

Scabies
Scabies is due to invasion of the epidermis by a mite (Acarus scabiei). It is acquired by direct contact with an affected person. It is most commonly transmitted between members of a family. The mite burrows along the skin causing a papular rash. The most commonly affected areas are the hands and wrists. Other areas include the soles of the feet, elbows, buttocks, axillae and genitalia.

Intense irritation occurs and is worse at night. Scratching may be followed by secondary bacterial infection. Treatment involves bathing followed by an application of benzyl benzoate lotion to the whole body. This procedure is repeated the following day. Clean clothes should be worn and the bed clothes changed.

Careful explanation is necessary, as the whole family should be treated whether they are itching or not.

Lice
Three different types of louse may affect the body. These are the head louse, the body louse and the pubic louse.

The head louse is common, particularly amongst school children. Nits are seen on the hair shaft and itching may occur.

Treatment involves application of malathion lotion (Prioderm) followed 12 hours later by shampooing and combing out the nits. This procedure is repeated after seven days.

Body lice are usually seen only in vagrants. Eggs are found in the seams of clothing. Itching occurs and scratch marks are seen. Treatment involves application of gamma benzene hexachloride lotion (Quellada) after the patient has bathed. Clean clothes should be worn. The contaminated clothing should be autoclaved.

Pubic lice cause intense itching in the genital area. Spread is by sexual contact. Treatment is with gamma benzene hexachloride shampoo (Lorexane).

Urticaria

Urticaria is an eruption of transient, circumscribed oedematous and itchy swellings which last only a few hours. Nettle stings, insect bites and jelly-fish stings cause local urticaria. Acute widespread urticaria can be seen in penicillin reactions, radiotherapy and autoimmune disease. Joint swelling and fever accompany intense irritation. Treatment of acute urticaria involves administration of an antihistamine drug, e.g. promethazine hydrochloride (Phenergan) or chlorpheniramine (Piriton). If swelling of the tongue and glottis occur together with signs of shock, adrenaline may be required. Intravenous hydrocortisone, a steroid, may also be necessary.

Psoriasis

Psoriasis is a common skin condition presenting as raised red plaques covered by silvery scales. The cause is unknown, although hereditary factors may play a part. Epidermal cell formation is increased and the increased blood supply causes oedema.

Medical and nursing problems
Sharply demarcated red plaques covered with silvery scales
— pattern varies
— lesions on knees and elbows are common
Pitting of fingernails
Broken nails
Scalp lesions

Arthritis
— about 7% are affected
Stress
Self-consciousness

Medical treatment

- Local treatment involves tar baths, ultraviolet light, and application of dithranol in Lassar's paste to the lesions.
- A weak steroid cream may be used to treat the face and flexures.
- Psoriasis of the scalp is treated with coal tar shampoo, and application of a tar and salicylic acid compound.
- Arthritis is treated with an anti-inflammatory drug such as ibuprofen (Brufen) or indomethacin (Indocid).
- Severe psoriasis may be treated with methotrexate. This is a folic acid antagonist which inhibits cell division (an antimitotic). It may depress bone marrow activity.
- Ultraviolet light is an effective form of treatment. A drug, 8-methoxypsoralen, is given two hours before treatment. Treatment is carried out three times per week. The patient should wear sunglasses from the time he takes the tablets until the time he retires at night.

Nursing intervention

- Gloves should be worn when applying dithranol. It is applied to the lesions only and is dusted with zinc and starch powder. Tubular gauze dressings are then applied. It can be removed the following day with light liquid paraffin.
- Dithranol should not be used on the face or in the flexures.
- Psoriasis may improve with rest and relaxation alone. Whilst he is in hospital, the patient is able to meet people with similar skin conditions. He should be advised to join the Psoriasis Association.
- The nurse should teach the patient to apply the cream to himself effectively.

Tumours of the skin

The most common malignant tumours of the skin are basal cell carcinoma and squamous cell carcinoma.

A basal cell carcinoma (rodent ulcer) is a slow-growing pearly nodule, which commonly occurs on the face or neck. Most occur after the age of 50 years. If left untreated, ulceration and local invasion occur. Treatment is with biopsy, radiotherapy or surgical excision.

A squamous cell carcinoma arises as a heaped-up nodule which may later ulcerate. Metastases may occur with this type of tumour. Treatment is similar to that for a basal cell carcinoma.

Varicose ulcers

Varicose ulcers of the legs occur in people who have disorders of venous drainage. Impairment of drainage may result from obstruction of veins by thrombosis or from incompetent valves in the veins.

Medical and nursing problems
Pigmentation
— along the line of the varicose veins
— around the ankles
Eczema
— erythema
— scaling
Oedema of ankles
Ulceration
— after minor injury

Medical treatment
- Local treatment involves thorough cleaning of the ulcer with a solution of eusol or sodium hypochlorite (Milton).
- An occlusive bandage of zinc paste or coal tar may be applied and left in position for one week.
- Skin grafts may be used on extensive granulating areas.

Nursing intervention
- Elastic stockings are helpful in the reduction of ankle oedema.
- If the patient is obese he should be encouraged to reduce weight.
- Walking is encouraged.
- The legs are elevated when resting.

Further reading

Nursing 2 (1983) *Skin* Volumes 9 and 10 (January and February).
Pegum, J.S. & Baker, H. (1979) *Dermatology*, 3rd edition. London: Baillière Tindall.
Sneddon, J.B. & Church, R.E. (1983) *Practical Dermatology*, 4th edition. London: Edward Arnold.
Wilkinson, O.S. (1977) *The Nursing and Management of Skin Diseases*, 4th edition. London: Faber & Faber.

14
Neuromedical Nursing

The nervous system is the control and communication system of the body. It is responsible for receiving and interpreting the messages which the body receives from its environment, for conscious sensation, and for control of motor activity. Disorders of the nervous system manifest themselves by changes in motor control, sensory perception, in consciousness or in behaviour.

Nerve tissue

Nerve tissue is made up of millions of nerve cells or neurones and their processes. These are the functional unit of the nervous system and are supported by connective tissue cells called glial cells.

Neurones

Nerve cells vary in size and shape but each has a cell body which contains a nucleus embedded in protoplasm. Each neurone has many processes: the short ones are called dendrites and the long process is called the axon or nerve fibre (Figure 50).

Impulses are transmitted from one neurone to another by the passage of a small electrical current down the axon from the cell body. This is produced by the movement of sodium and potassium ions across the membrane of the axon. When the current reaches the end of the axon, a neurotransmitter chemical is released. These chemicals cross the synapse between the processes of the cells and either stimulate or inhibit the next cell in producing its own electrical current.

In some neurones, the axon is insulated by a myelin membrane. In order that impulses may be transmitted along myelinated nerve fibres, the myelin sheath is absent at certain points known as the nodes of Ranvier (Figure 50). The impulses pass from one node of Ranvier to the next.

White matter refers to aggregations of myelinated axons from many neurones, supported by neurological cells. The lipid

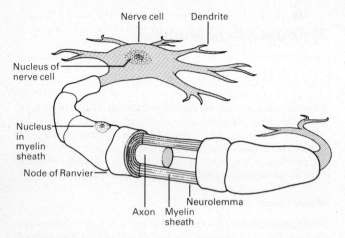

Figure 50. A neurone.

substance myelin has a whitish colour that gives the white matter its name.

Grey matter is the part of the nervous system which contains either nerve cell bodies and dendrites or bundles of unmyelinated axons and neurological cells.

The nervous system

The nervous system is composed of the central nervous system, the peripheral nervous system and the autonomic nervous system.

The central nervous system

The central nervous system comprises the brain and the spinal cord.

The brain can be anatomically divided into three parts: the cerebrum, the cerebellum and the brain stem (which includes the midbrain, the pons and the medulla oblongata). The brain occupies the interior of the skull and is continuous with the spinal cord at the foramen magnum (the hole in the base of the skull through which the spinal cord passes).

The spinal cord runs in the spinal canal from the foramen magnum to the level of the first lumbar vertebra. Although anatomically the spinal cord is a continuous structure, it is convenient to divide the cord into eight cervical, twelve thoracic, five lumbar, five sacral and one coccygeal segment. Each segment receives sensory (afferent) nerve roots and gives off motor (efferent) nerve roots on either side. These nerve roots join together to form peripheral nerves which pass out between the vertebrae.

The brain and the spinal cord are covered by protective membranes called meninges. There are three layers:

Dura mater — outer layer
Arachnoid mater — middle layer
Pia mater — inner layers

The peripheral nervous system

The peripheral nervous system comprises the cranial nerves which arise from or travel to the brain stem and the spinal nerves which arise from or travel to the spinal cord. These fibres are myelinated and can be classified as motor or sensory nerves. The motor nerves innervate voluntary muscle throughout the body. The sensory nerves carry messages from the sense organs to the central nervous system.

The autonomic nervous system

The autonomic nervous system comprises the sympathetic system and the para-sympathetic system. The nerve fibres of these systems are non-myelinated and are concerned mainly with the control of involuntary muscle. They consist largely of efferent neurones: motor fibres supplying the involuntary muscles in the walls of organs such as the stomach, intestines, bladder, heart and blood vessels, and secretory fibres supplying organs such as the liver, pancreas and kidney.

Investigations

Plain X-rays

Skull, spinal and chest X-rays may be performed.

Electroencephalography (EEG)

The electrical activity of the brain can be measured and compared with a normal pattern.

Lumbar puncture

A lumbar puncture is frequently performed in neurological diseases:

> To remove a sample of cerebrospinal fluid (CSF) for diagnostic purposes
> To estimate and perhaps reduce cerebrospinal pressure
> To give drugs (intrathecal injections)
> To introduce radiological contrast

A needle is usually inserted between the third and fourth lumbar vertebrae so as to prevent damage to the spinal cord. Following the procedure the patient is advised to lie flat to prevent headaches which may develop due to low pressure. It is also important to encourage a fluid intake of 200 ml hourly to help the formation of cerebrospinal fluid.

Computerized axial tomography (CAT scan, CT scan)

This is an invaluable non-invasive investigation which involves a series of X-ray tomograms cutting through the brain from the occiput upwards. The contents of the skull are visualized and a computerized assessment can be made of the density of the structures X-rayed. This technique has largely superseded cerebral angiography and pneumoencephalography.

Cerebral angiography

The cerebral blood vessels can be shown by injecting a radio-opaque contrast medium into the carotid artery. This investigation can be performed under general anaesthesia. It is important to observe the puncture site and monitor the neurological state of the person for six to eight hours following this procedure.

Pneumoencephalography

This investigation is used to detect tumours close to the ventricular system and certain degenerative disorders. Air or a radio-opaque solution is introduced via a cannula into a lateral ventricle or into the subarachnoid space. Following this procedure, it is important that the patient's conscious level is observed as air could become trapped in the ventricles, causing drowsiness and coma.

Myelography

A myelogram is a radiological examination in which a contrast solution is used to outline the subarachnoid space, the spinal cord and its nerve roots. It is used to delineate tumours of the spine and prolapsed intervertebral discs. The patient will have to lie flat or sit upright according to which contrast medium is used.

Visual field testing

The nerve fibres from the retina of the eye pass through the optic nerves, the optic chiasma and the optic tracts to the visual cortex in the occipital lobe. Changes in the integrity of this pathway may lead to defects in the patient's field of vision.

Electromyography (EMG)

Electrical activity occurs within muscle fibres and can be detected by needle electrodes inserted into the muscles.

Neurological assessment

Neurological assessment of the patient by the nurse is of vital importance. Recognition of change in a patient's condition depends on serial observations and the nurse is in a position to perform this degree of monitoring. The aim of assessment is twofold: first, to discover any deterioration or improvement in a patient's condition so that medical intervention can be made if necessary; second, to aid in the discovery of which area of the nervous system is involved. The nurse's assessment is recorded on a neurological observation chart (Figure 51).

Conscious level

The patient's conscious level gives an indication of the general functioning of the brain. The patient should be woken if necessary and his degree of alertness ascertained. It is important to record the patient's conscious level in a way that cannot be

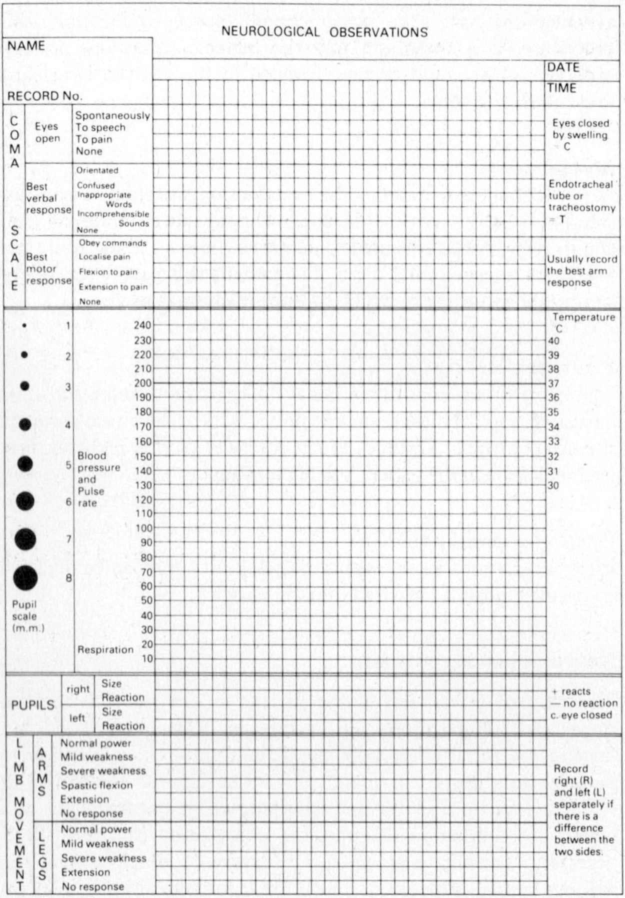

Figure 51. Neurological observation chart.

misinterpreted. To say a patient is 'semi-conscious' is unhelpful, as it could mean he is drowsy or nearly unconscious. Level of consciousness can be rated on a coma scale which gives specific information. This scale is in three sections: his eye response, his best verbal response and his best motor response (see Figure 51).

Pupil response
When examining the pupils the following should be noted:
  equality of the pupils
  size of the pupils
  reaction of the pupils to light

Any inequality in the size of the pupils should be noted. Some people with asymmetrical faces normally have unequal pupils, so it is important to have noted whether the pupils are equal or unequal in size when *initially* assessing a patient.

The reaction to light is tested by bringing a strong light with a narrow beam rapidly towards the pupil. If the third cranial nerve is functioning, the pupil should constrict briskly. When the light is shone into one eye, the pupil of the other eye should also constrict briskly; this is called a consensual reflex.

Limb movements
Paresis (weakness) or plegia (paralysis) of a limb is an important sign. It may indicate a lesion of the opposite cerebral hemisphere, in which case both limbs on one side may be affected; this condition is known as hemiparesis or hemiplegia. When both legs are affected, it is termed paraparesis or paraplegia. If all limbs are involved, this is known as quadriparesis or quadriplegia.

To test for arm weakness, the patient is asked to squeeze the nurse's fingers. If he squeezes each of the nurse's hands with each of his hands at the same time the nurse may feel some difference in strength, but this may be inaccurate as the right hand is often stronger in right-handed people. One other method is to ask the patient to hold both arms straight out in front of him and to shut his eyes. After a short period the weak arm will waver or gradually fall downwards.

Ideally, leg movement is tested by watching the patient walk, when one foot or leg may be seen to drag. If the patient is unable to get up or move his legs when asked, a stimulus is applied, e.g. pressing with the top of a pen on the leg, to note whether the limb is withdrawn or extended. Power can be tested by asking the patient to push against pressure applied by the nurse; for example, after the patient has raised his leg, he attempts to keep it raised while the nurse presses down on it.

Vital signs
Blood pressure, pulse and temperature are recorded. These may be

of secondary importance in detecting change, as level of consciousness and pupillary reaction may give more rapid information.

The advantages of one nurse repeatedly carrying out this assessment over a period of time is self-evident. However, with shorter shifts, changes in the nurse caring for a particular patient are inevitable. Whenever possible, the nurse taking over should assess the patient with the nurse who has been caring for him, in order that continuity of assessment is maintained.

DISORDERS OF THE BRAIN AND SPINAL CORD

Cerebrovascular disease

The brain receives its blood from the two internal carotid and the two vertebral arteries. The two systems are linked together by the circle of Willis (Figure 52).

Approximately a fifth of the cardiac output usually passes through the carotid and vertebral arteries to supply the intracranial structures.

The three main causes of reduced blood supply to the brain are vascular:

    cerebral haemorrhage
    cerebral thrombosis
    cerebral embolism

The brain is damaged due to a reduction in the amount of oxygen reaching it. Occlusion of a cerebral artery will normally lead to infarction (death) in the tissues it supplies. Conditions caused in this way are known as cerebrovascular accidents or 'strokes'.

Cerebral haemorrhage

Primary cerebral haemorrhage is associated with hypertension and arteriosclerosis. It usually presents abruptly. The patient complains of a violent headache and there may be a history of physical exertion prior to the onset. In over half the patients there is a loss of consciousness, sometimes accompanied by an epileptic fit. A large haemorrhage coupled with a loss of consciousness has a

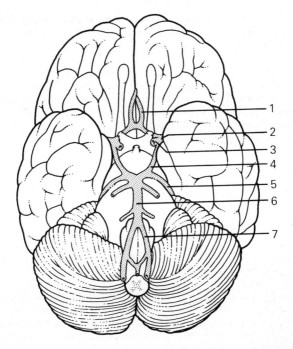

Figure 52. The circle of Willis. 1, anterior cerebral artery; 2, middle cerebral artery; 3, internal carotid artery; 4, posterior communicating artery; 5, posterior cerebral artery; 6, basilar artery; 7, vertebral artery.

poor prognosis; approximately half the patients die within a few days.

Cerebral thrombosis
Atheromatous changes (patchy degeneration in the walls of large arteries in which fat-like plaques appear) are often present in the cerebral arteries of people over 60 years of age. However, even quite extensive atheroma may be symptomless. Atheromatous plaques associated with arteriosclerosis can cause blockage of the vessel lumen. This reduces the amount of oxygen reaching the part

of the brain supplied by the diseased vessel. Infarction may then occur.

Occlusion due to cerebral thrombosis may affect any of the branches of the circle of Willis, but the most commonly involved are the internal carotid and middle cerebral arteries. These supply the motor and sensory areas of the cerebrum and the internal capsule within the temporal and frontal lobes. The most common feature is hemiplegia. Speech may be affected if the dominant hemisphere (containing the speech centre) is involved.

Cerebral embolism

An embolus may block the cerebral blood vessels. It normally occurs suddenly, when an embolus has broken off from the heart or from atheromatous plaques in the large arteries in the neck and thorax. The symptoms and signs of an infarction due to an embolus are similar to those due to thrombosis.

Assessment of the patient

The picture a patient presents varies considerably, and depends on the site and extent of the infarction. As the patient may be unconscious, it is important to obtain as much information as possible from those present at the time concerning the onset and development of symptoms.

Some of the areas in assessing a patient that need to be considered are:

1 *Level of consciousness.* May range from an unconscious to conscious state.

2 *Degree of paralysis.* Hemiplegia or hemiparesis may be present. Paralysis of the face and arm, but not of the leg, can occur.

3 *Speech.* Absence of speech (aphasia) or difficulty with speech (dysphasia) may be present.

4 *Age.* Patients are usually elderly, but this disease can occur in patients aged 40 to 60 years. It is extremely rare below this age group.

5 *Onset.* This varies from gradual to sudden.

6 *Previous medical history.* There may be no relevant past medical history, or the patient may have previous problems such as hypertension or heart failure.

Medical treatment

Medical treatment is based on correcting or stabilizing any underlying problems which may have contributed to the cerebrovascular accident. However, as has been stated, there may have been no obvious previous medical problem. The commonest diseases which may need treatment are heart failure and hypertension. Diuretic, cardiac and hypotensive drugs may be required.

Nursing intervention

- The care of the patient will vary according to the extent of the cerebrovascular accident.
- If a patient is unconscious, the primary aim is to protect him from the dangers of unconsciousness and immobility. For care of the unconscious patient, see page 32.

Care of a patient with hemiplegia:

- The aim of care is to achieve the fullest degree of independence possible.
- Rehabilitation should be begun as soon as the patient is conscious to ensure the maximum degree of recovery. It will be performed by a group of people which, in addition to the nursing and medical staff, includes the physiotherapist, the occupational therapist and the social worker.
- Paralysis is flaccid at first, but may become spastic as muscle tone returns. Positioning is therefore important to prevent development of contractures (Figure 53).
- The physiotherapist will teach and supervise a range of exercises aimed at preventing the patient from neglecting his paralysed side.
- The degree to which a patient will, and is encouraged to, use his paralysed side is often the key factor in the degree of independence achieved.
- Certain aids for walking, such as a Zimmer frame, tripod or walking stick, may be required.
- It is vital for the nurse to observe the patient's feet as, if the toes point down, foot drop may develop. This would make walking very difficult, if not impossible. Sand bags are sometimes used to keep the foot in the correct position, or ocasionally light splinting of the foot and ankle may be necessary.

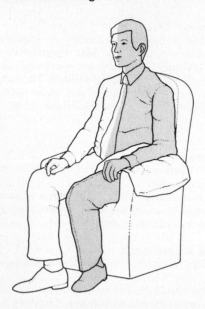

Figure 53. Supporting a patient with a left hemiplegia in a chair.

- The nurse, in conjunction with the occupational therapist, has an important role in encouraging the patient's independence. The patient should be encouraged to wash, feed and dress himself. The aim is to instruct, supervise and support the patient carrying out these activities, rather than performing them for him.
- The occupational therapist will be particularly involved in assessing the patient's disabilities and teaching him ways to overcome them.
- As the patient's independence returns, the occupational therapist will help supervise activities such as getting in and out of the bath, dressing, feeding and cooking. She may provide aids such as adapted cutlery, non-stick mats, plate guards and aids to bathing.
- The social worker and occupational therapist, in conjunction with the family, will be involved in assessing the home

situation to ensure any problems the patient will have within his home are overcome.

Care of a patient with dysphasia:
- The speech therapist has an important part to play in helping a patient with any difficulties with speech he may have.
- A patient with dysphasia may be able to think rationally, but not express himself verbally. This can cause tremendous frustration, depression and anger, and underlines the importance of psychological nursing care.

Psychological support:
- The loss of independence that occurs after a cerebrovascular accident causes considerable distress and frustration.
- The patient may be unable to, or find it difficult to, wash himself or eat or drink on his own; he may be incontinent of urine or faeces and may be acutely aware of his paralysed side.
- Dysphasia can cause immense feeling of anger and impotence because of difficulties in communication. There may be a tendency for people to treat him as 'simple' or as a child — both in terms of their actions and their language.
- The resultant loss of self-esteem, depression and frustration can cause serious problems.
- The patient must be treated as an intelligent adult.
- If incontinence occurs, or help is required with feeding, an understanding of how it feels to be helpless may ease the distress. One must emphasize verbally how difficult it must be for the patient.
- An assurance that many aspects of independence will return is important.
- A nurse must be continually aware how the patient may be feeling about his helplessness and lack of independence. Consequently her speech and nursing care will reflect that understanding and thereby help maintain her patient's dignity and self-respect.

Multiple sclerosis

Multiple, or disseminated, sclerosis is one of the most common of the nervous diseases. The cause is unknown. The myelin sheath of the neurone disintegrates and therefore the nerve is no longer able to conduct impulses correctly. This leads to impairment of the function of the area supplied by the nerve. A striking feature of this condition is its tendency to undergo remissions and relapses; thus the disease may take years to develop.

Medical and nursing problems

Multiple sclerosis can affect the nerves throughout the brain and spinal cord, so the patients can present with a variety of signs. However, with each consecutive attack, the neurological impairment increases and the patient will eventually become chronically disabled.

Common early signs:

Visual disturbances
— unilateral optic neuritis is often the first sign
— blurring of vision
— double vision
— pain on movement of eye
Sensations of numbness or tingling in a limb
Weakness of a limb
— common in lower limb with dragging of foot
— can involve arm
    loss of power
    inability to perform fine movements with hand
Impaired control of bladder function
— urgency of micturition
— incontinenence

Later signs:

Spastic paraplegia
— walking becomes difficult as spasticity of legs increases
— aids such as a walking frame may be needed
— a wheelchair may be required
Ataxia
— due to cerebellar and brain stem lesions
— coordination of hand movements difficult and characterized by a jerkiness (intention tremor)
— irregular and jerky movements of lower limb may occur
Disturbance of speech

— takes a variety of forms
— may be slurred and irregular, with syllables pronounced separately (staccato or scanning speech)
Mood disturbance
— varies from euphoria to irritability and depression
Loss of control of bladder and bowel function
— incontinence of faeces or constipation
Mystagmus
— involuntary rapid movements of the eye

Medical treatment

- There is no specific treatment for multiple sclerosis.
- Drugs may be given — the commonest of which is adrenocorticotrophic hormone (ACTH). Its benefit remains unproven.
- Urinary tract infections are common and are treated with the appropriate antibiotic.
- Rest is required during an acute exacerbation.

Nursing intervention

The aim of care is to help the patient achieve a maximum degree of physical independence and psychological adjustment to his condition. In the early stages of multiple sclerosis, when it becomes clear that disabilities are developing, care is directed at supporting the patient and his family and educating them about the nature of the disease. This section will be confined to the care of a patient in the later stages when paraplegia has occurred.

Environment:
- Wherever possible a person should be cared for at home. Certain changes may be required to accommodate a wheelchair and to aid independence, e.g. doors may need to be widened, alterations within the bathroom and lavatory may be required, or a ramp may be needed to the front door.
- Support within this environment is vital and can be provided by community nurses, general practitioners and social workers.
- If the family and home situation is unsuitable, the person may need to be cared for in a community nursing home.

- Admissions to hospital may become necessary due to an exacerbation of the disease or a particular physical problem such as a urinary tract infection.

Problems with elimination:
- Bladder care is required, as micturition is often impaired. As bladder control deteriorates, incontinence can occur, with the subsequent likelihood of urinary tract infections.
- Catheterization on a long-term basis may be required. For men, a sheath placed over the penis and attached to a drainage bag is sometimes used.
- Bowel care is established according to the individual and his environment. A high roughage diet, a good fluid intake and regular aperients may be required. Some patients cannot evacuate faeces and may need suppositories or an enema before manual evacuation.

Problems with impaired independence:
- There will be a number of activities with which the person may require assistance.
- He may require assistance with bathing and maintaining his personal hygiene.
- Help may be required with eating or providing food (shopping, cooking).
- Difficulty in washing and drying, immobility and incontinence all make sore or broken skin possible. Changing position (the patient may be able to do this by lifting himself up using the arms of a wheelchair), care in washing and drying if incontinent and a nutritious diet will help maintain healthy skin.

Problems due to visual impairment:
- Nurses must remember that a person with multiple sclerosis may have difficulty with his vision. Such an awareness can prevent embarrassment or distress to the patient. Talking books (tape-recorded stories) can be provided.

Psychological care:
- Multiple sclerosis patients have an image of being 'bed-ridden and crippled'. It is important for the nurse to help the person

realize that this image is too simple. She should assist people to concentrate on maintaining their independence according to their particular disabilities.

- The fact that this disease is progressive means that psychological support is critical. When independence achieved after a hard struggle is diminished by progression of the disease, it can cause despair and dependency.
- It may help the individual to join the multiple sclerosis society.
- See also page 237.

Epilepsy

Nerve cells function by discharging small electrical impulses. If the brain cells suddenly produce an abnormal burst of electrical impulses, an epileptic fit may result. Patients who have repeated fits are said to suffer from epilepsy. Loss or impairment of consciousness frequently occurs in association with an attack, but the abnormal electrical discharge may involve certain limited areas of the brain without interfering with the level of consciousness.

There are four main types of attack — major (grand mal), minor (petit mal), temporal lobe epilepsy and jacksonian epilepsy.

Varieties of epilepsy

Idiopathic epilepsy. This is where there is no apparent organic damage to account for the epileptic attacks. They normally start in the early years of life and there appears to be a hereditary tendency.

Symptomatic epilepsy. This is where there is organic damage to explain the attack. Such damage may be caused by a cerebral tumour or head injury, or may be due to abuse of alcohol or other drugs.

Investigations

The purpose of investigating a patient with epilepsy is to discover whether there is a cause which can be treated, apart from the symptomatic treatment of the epilepsy itself. Electroencephalography (EEG) is the main investigation performed. Other neurological investigations will be performed if a cerebral tumour is thought to be present.

Grand mal (major epilepsy)

A grand mal fit is a generalized attack which may be idiopathic or symptomatic in origin. It comprises four stages: the aura, the tonic phase, the clonic phase and the post-epileptic coma.

1   The aura

An aura is a warning and may take a variety of forms; for example, epigastric sensations, vertigo, or feelings of fear. The aura can last from a few seconds to half a minute and may give the patient enough time to anticipate the fit and so be able to move himself away from obvious danger. However, not all patients have an aura.

Nursing intervention
- The patient is laid on the floor and an area around him is cleared of furniture or objects on which he may damage himself.
- Dentures are removed and a rolled handkerchief or piece of cloth is placed between the teeth. Spectacles are also removed.
- As the aura may not occur or may be of a short duration, it may not be possible to perform these actions.
- Once the tonic phase has started no attempt should be made to force the mouth open to insert a gag. Such an attempt can result in severe damage to the teeth or the muscles of the jaw, or a fracture of the lower jaw can occur.

2   The tonic phase

The patient often cries out as he loses consciousness. All his muscles contract. His arms flex and his legs extend. As the muscles involved in respiration are affected, the patient will become cyanosed. This phase will last from about 5 to 30 seconds.

Nursing intervention
Tight clothing around the neck, chest and waist should be loosened.

3   The clonic phase

This is the convulsive stage during which muscles repeatedly relax and contract, sometimes violently. There may be incontinence. After about two minutes the convulsing gradually ceases and the patient lapses into a flaccid coma.

Nursing intervention
- The convulsive movements of the limbs should not be restrained as this can cause severe damage. It is worth ensuring again that there is sufficient free space around the patient.

4   The post-epileptic coma

The muscles relax and the respirations become stertorous (snoring sound). Flushing of the face may occur. This period may last for a short interval or for several hours. The patient's level of consciousness improves and he then passes through a transient period of disorientation. This is followed by a period of normal sleep.

Nursing intervention
- Maintenance of a clear airway is essential. The patient needs to be positioned as one would an unconscious patient. Removal of excessive secretions from the mouth and pharynx may be necessary.
- If incontinence of urine and faeces has occurred, clothing will need to be changed and the skin cleaned.
- The patient and other people present are reassured.
- The patient is observed to ensure he is returning to a normal state and that post-epileptic automatism is not present. This is where automatic acts occur following an epileptic attack of which he has no knowledge. These acts may consist of wandering around, dressing and undressing or other embarrassing and/or dangerous behaviours. If this occurs, the patient may need to be restrained or have someone with him until he is fully orientated.

Patients suffering a grand mal seizure do not necessarily pass through all the stages described. There is considerable individual variation in the way a grand mal seizure manifests itself.

Petit mal (minor epilepsy)

Petit mal epilepsy is idiopathic and usually begins in childhood. It takes the form of momentary alterations of consciousness, so that the patient may, for example, pause in conversation, have a vacant expression, or suddenly stop while walking. The problems of such attacks is that they may occur in a place which may be dangerous, for example in the bath or in the middle of the road.

Temporal lobe epilepsy

In fits caused by lesions in or near the temporal lobe, the aura, which is always prominent, may be the sole feature or the attack may progress to a generalized convulsion.

A wide variety of sensory and motor disturbances may occur. Sensory disturbances take the form of hallucinations of smell, taste and perception. The latter is known as the *déjà vu* phenomenon — a feeling that what is happening has happened before. Motor disturbances are equally varied. The patient looks dazed and does not respond normally when questioned. Aggressive behaviour occasionally occurs.

Jacksonian or focal epilepsy

Jacksonian epilepsy is a convulsion originating in the precentral motor cortex. This is the area of the brain which lies immediately in front of the motor cortex and is responsible for some gross postural movements. The attack starts in one part of the body and is either limited to this area, or spreads, when it may progress to a major convulsion. One common pattern is for a convulsion to begin with the thumb or finger and the corner of the mouth. It progresses down that side of the body and may then involve the opposite limbs in a generalized fit, with loss of consciousness.

Observation of a seizure

It is evident from the above descriptions that there is a wide variety of epileptic fits in terms of the degree of loss of consciousness and the form of sensory and motor disturbances.

Following a seizure a nurse may be required to fill in a questionnaire about the fit so as to aid diagnosis and monitor the effectiveness of treatment. The following list is a guide to the questions asked, but other unusual features may occur and should be noted:

What was the patient doing prior to the attack?
Did the patient let out a cry?
Did he lose consciousness? If so, for how long?
If convulsions occurred, where did they start?
Did they spread to any other part of the body?
Was the patient incontinent of urine or faeces?
Were any injuries sustained?
How long did the fit last?
What was the patient's pattern of behaviour following recovery?

Drug treatment

Certain drugs have been found to diminish the severity and frequency of epileptic attacks, and in some cases to abolish them completely. Anticonvulsant drugs are thought to act by increasing the stability of the neuronal membranes by altering the electrochemical ion permeability. This prevents the spread of the abnormal brain activity.

Perseverance in treatment is essential, as the patient must continue to take anticonvulsant drugs for at least two years after an attack if a relapse is to be avoided.

Some of the commoner drugs used are:
phenobarbitone (60–300 mg/day)
phenytoin (150–600 mg/day)
primidone (125–1500 mg/day)
sodium valproate (600–2600 mg/day)
clonazepam (1–8 mg/day)

Some patients may require a combination of two anticonvulsant drugs.

Advice for a patient with epilepsy

People with epilepsy can easily be overprotected. A fit can cause considerable alarm and distress to the patient and especially to those present. Consequently there is a tendency to cocoon the patient and thereby make him feel very different. It is important that the patient, his family, and those he works with are helped to accept the epilepsy and taught how to manage a fit. This will help to allow the patient to lead as normal a life as possible. However, certain restrictions are necessary if the individual is to manage his epilepsy safely.

It is important that drugs are taken at the prescribed times. They must be taken for a number of years even if an epileptic attack has not occurred. Alcohol may have to be restricted or forbidden as it increases the sedative effect of some anticonvulsant drugs such as phenobarbitone.

If the epilepsy is not well controlled, advice will be necessary to ensure the patient does not undertake activities during which a fit would be particularly dangerous. Examples of such activities are smoking when alone, sports such as cycling or swimming, having a bath (a shower is preferable), and working with certain types of machinery. Many of these, and similar activities, are safe if the individual is accompanied.

There are legal restrictions to driving. In Britain, a person suffering from epilepsy may only hold a driving licence if he has not had an epileptic attack while awake for three years. It does not matter whether he is or is not taking anticonvulsant drugs. This only applies to private cars and not to heavy goods or public service vehicles.

A patient in Britain should be made aware of the British Epilepsy Association, from whom he can obtain an identity card which states he suffers from epilepsy. The point of this card is that, should a seizure occur outside the home, people will understand what is happening and the appropriate care can be given.

Status epilepticus

In status epilepticus, attacks follow each other without the patient regaining consciousness. It is a grave emergency and admission to hospital is necessary. Management involves stopping the cycle of fits by the use of intravenous drugs such as diazepam, maintaining a clear airway, and preventing injury. Full care of the unconscious patient is necessary. Padded cot sides will be required. A common precipitating factor in status epilepticus is when a patient suddenly stops taking his anticonvulsant drugs.

Parkinson's disease (paralysis agitans)

The extrapyramidal tract is concerned with the regulation of posture and the performance of habitual and automatic movements which form the background to the skilled, purposeful activities of daily life. It consists of nerve fibres arising from the cortex, the cerebellum and the basal ganglia.

Parkinson's disease is due to the degeneration of those neurones in the brain stem and basal ganglia which contain dopamine. The cause of this degeneration is unknown. This process usually begins between the ages of 50 and 60 years.

In Parkinson's disease the level of dopamine in the corpus striatum, which is the major centre in the extrapyramidal tract, is severely reduced. Research has also shown that the level of the chemical transmitter acetylcholine within the nervous system is increased. The signs and symptoms of this disease are due to this imbalance of chemical transmitters.

Medical and nursing problems
Tremor
— involuntary
— usually begins in one upper limb
— later involves lower limb on same side
— other side then affected in upper limb
— hand is most affected in upper limb
    movement at metacarpophalangeal joints
    movement of thumb
    when combined termed 'pill-rolling' movement
Muscular rigidity
— most evident on passive flexion and extension of wrist
— movement jerky due to superimposed tremor (cog-wheel rigidity)
Facial changes
— facial mobility impaired
— mask-like appearance
— doesn't alter easily in response to emotion
— staring appearance to eyes
— spontaneous ocular movements (uncommon)
Disorders of movement
— power slightly impaired

— movements performed very slowly (bradykinesia)
— hands particularly affected, e.g.
  clumsiness
  difficulty writing
  difficulty using cutlery
  difficulty fastening buttons
Gait
— swinging of arms diminished, then lost
— slow, shuffling, small steps
— may be 'festinating' (hurrying with small steps, as if trying to catch up with his centre of gravity)
— difficulty starting to walk and stopping
Speech
— slurred and monotonous
— sentences may become an unintelligible run of words
Salivation
— excessive salivation may occur

Medical treatment

- Drugs are given to reduce tremor, rigidity and bradykinesia. These drugs can be divided into those which increase the concentration of dopamine in the basal ganglia and those which antagonize the activity of acetylcholine.
- Drugs used to lessen rigidity and tremor are benzhexol (2 mg four times daily) and orphenadrine hydrochloride (50 mg three times daily).
- The main drug used to reduce bradykinesia and rigidity is levodopa. This is converted to dopamine in the brain. Its use may be hampered due to its side-effects and it may need to be replaced by other drugs such as bromocriptine, or carbidopa may be used. Carbidopa consists of levodopa plus a dopa-decarboxylase inhibitor, which makes side-effects less likely.
- Stereotaxic surgery, such as thalamotomy, may be required to treat the tremor.

Nursing intervention

- Drugs are given as prescribed with or after food.
- Side-effects of drugs must be monitored. Levodopa causes nausea and vomiting, postural hypotension, confusion and

jerky, involuntary (choreo-athetoid) movements. Benzhexol and orphenadrine hydrochloride can cause confusion, gastrointestinal disturbances and urinary retention.

- Postural hypotension is detected by monitoring the blood pressure lying and standing twice daily.
- The patient may require help with initiating movement. He may need to be rocked backwards and forwards to start walking.
- The patient may also need help with activities involving fine movement, such as writing, doing up buttons or using cutlery.
- Assurance and support are necessary to lessen depressive feelings due to the range of disabilities, poor self-image and social isolation.

Infections

Infections may involve the membranes of the brain (meningitis), the substance of the brain (encephalitis), or the spinal cord (myelitis). Meningoencephalitis or meningoencephalomyelitis may occur, particularly in viral infections.

Meningitis

Acute meningitis (or more accurately acute leptomeningitis) is inflammation of the pia mater and arachnoid, which inevitably involves the subarachnoid space and cerebrospinal fluid (CSF). Infection reaches the meninges in three main ways: through a fracture of the skull, extension to the meninges of a pre-existing pyogenic infection of one of the nasal sinuses, the middle ear or mastoid, or via the bloodstream.

Any pathogenic organism can cause this disease once the subarachnoid space has been penetrated, but the commonest are meningococci, the pneumococci, streptococci and staphylococci. Many viral infections such as measles and glandular fever are associated with a mild meningitis. Virus infections that mainly affect the meninges mostly belong to the enterovirus group.

Medical and nursing problems
Headache
— usually the first sign

— increases in severity
— may be diffuse or frontal
— often radiates down the neck into the back
Fever
— normally 38–40°C
Photophobia (intolerance to light)
Neck stiffness
— neck cannot be flexed so as to bring the chin down
   onto the chest due to spasm of the extensor muscles of
   the neck
Kernig's sign may be present
— an attempt to passively extend the knee with the hip fully
   flexed causes spasm of the hamstring muscles and pain
Vomiting
— especially in the early stages
Convulsions
— common in children
— rare in adults
Changes in level of consciousness
— if infection is severe
— drowsy
— irritable
— delirious
— may lapse into a coma if untreated

Medical investigation and treatment
- A lumbar puncture and examination of the CSF will be
  performed to aid in the diagnosis.
- Antibiotics are given. Penicillin in high doses is the antibiotic
  commonly used in meningococcal and pneumococcal
  meningitis. It is given intramuscularly, intravenously or
  occasionally intrathecally. Different antibiotics may be given
  according to which organism is isolated from the CSF.
- Rehydration is necessary; intravenous fluid or fluid via a
  nasogastric tube is given.
- Lumbar punctures may be performed daily until the
  cerebrospinal fluid is sterile and the cell count normal.
- Analgesia is prescribed for headaches and may be given
  intramuscularly. These may be severe.
- Sedation may be prescribed if the patient is restless.

Nursing intervention
- Serial neurological observations are performed to assess the patient's level of consciousness.
- The patient is nursed in a darkened room due to the photophobia. Dark glasses may also help.
- Temperature recordings are performed hourly to monitor the pyrexia and the effectiveness of antibiotics.
- Analgesia is given three-hourly.
- If bacterial meningitis is present, the patient is barrier nursed to prevent cross-infection.
- Fluid intake and output are monitored to ensure rehydration is adequate.
- Assurance and support are given to reduce the fear, anxiety and loneliness caused by the disease, particularly if the patient needs to be isolated.

Encephalitis

Encephalitis (inflammation of the brain) is usually caused by a virus. Virus particles can reach the brain via the bloodstream or along the nerves, having first caused varying degrees of systemic disturbance. The severity of the disease varies according to the type of virus involved. Acute infections are usually caused by viruses that primarily invade the brain, such as in poliomyelitis or rabies. The herpes simplex virus is responsible for many of the severe forms of encephalitis occurring in Britain. Less serious forms of encephalitis occur in diseases such as measles or mumps, or occasionally occur as the result of a vaccination, e.g. rubella vaccination.

Medical and nursing problems
Headache
Mild fever
Confusion
Drowsiness
Convulsions, particularly in young children
Neck stiffness ⎫
Kernig's sign ⎬ may or may not be present

Medical investigation and treatment
- There is, as yet, no specific treatment for most types of encephalitis.
- Analgesia is given for headaches.
- Lumbar punctures are performed.
- Antiviral drugs such as cytosine arabinoside may be given.
- Anticonvulsants may be required.

Nursing intervention
- Observations for convulsions is important.
- Barrier nursing will be instituted.
- See also nursing intervention for meningitis (page 251).

Conclusion
Most patients with acute encephalitis recover, although some are left with permanent neurological or psychological damage.

Myelitis

Myelitis is inflammation of the spinal cord, normally involving both the grey and white matter. It may be due to a variety of causes, including bacterial infection (pyogenic or tuberculous), viral infection, and some forms of demyelinating disease. The poliovirus is an enterovirus which affects the cells of the somatic efferent columns. It is spread by the faecal–oral route and, although rare in Britain, is still present world-wide. Immunization with live, attenuated virus taken orally on a sugar lump is greatly reducing the world incidence of the disease.

Medical and nursing problems
Fever
Pain in the back
— often a marked feature
Paralysis of the trunk and lower limbs
Sensory loss
— may not be complete
Poor control or function of the bladder and bowel

Medical and nursing intervention
- If a specific cause can be determined, appropriate action can be taken. This often involves a course of antibiotic therapy. If an organism cannot be isolated, a course of broad-spectrum antibiotics is prescribed.
- Nursing intervention is based on the degree of paralysis; the full range of nursing care for someone with paraplegia may be necessary.
- The prognosis is dependent on the nature and severity of the infection. There may be a full recovery, but permanent paralysis may occur. Even if the disease remits, concern is still present as it may have been the first sign of multiple sclerosis.

DISEASES OF THE PERIPHERAL NERVES

Peripheral neuritis

Neuritis literally means the inflammation of a nerve, but the term is used generally to describe pain and impairment of the function of a peripheral nerve. The peripheral neuropathies are a large group of diseases which can be classified into two groups — acute and chronic.

Acute neuropathy

Acute neuropathies can be classified according to the cause into acute toxic polyneuritis, acute infectious polyneuritis, or acute post-infective polyneuritis (Guillain–Barré syndrome). They may follow infection with known viruses such as mumps and herpes zoster, may occur as an allergic response to tetanus serum, may result from glandular fever, or may be caused by porphyria (a disorder of haemoglobin metabolism in which episodes of haemoglobin breakdown occur).

Medical and nursing problems
Prior to developing weakness, the patient may have been in good health, although he may recall having had a cold or bout of 'flu.

Numbness and weakness in all limbs
— develops rapidly over 24 to 48 hours
— legs usually affected first
— weakness spreads up the body (ascending paralysis)
Weakness of muscles of swallowing and respiration
— in severe cases
Sensory loss
— in area of motor weakness
Disturbed bowel and bladder function

Medical treatment
- Respiratory function must be maintained. In severe cases artificial ventilation may be required.
- Infection is treated with antibiotics. Prophylactic antibiotics may be given to prevent a chest infection developing.
- Steroids may be prescribed, although their benefit is not proven.
- Intravenous fluid may be required to maintain an adequate fluid intake.
- Micturition may be aided by a urinary catheter as retention of urine is common.
- Physiotherapy is required to prevent joint stiffness and contractures developing.

Nursing intervention
- Respiratory rate and depth are monitored. Restlessness must be noted as it may mean cerebral hypoxia is occurring.
- Deep-breathing exercises are encouraged.
- Fluid output and input are recorded to monitor hydration.
- Bran, aperients or enemas may be required to maintain normal bowel actions.
- Passive limb movements are performed at least four times daily to prevent joint stiffness and contractures. Night splints may be required. Hydrotherapy may also be used. A bed cradle is advisable.
- Support and assurance are given to reduce the anxiety and fear caused by the loss of movement and the suddenness with which it has developed.
- The patient's skin is observed to ensure it is not becoming red or sore.

Conclusion

Acute peripheral neuropathy varies in its severity and course. In most patients, the weakness increases for one to two weeks, then remains stationary for two to four weeks before a gradual recovery takes place. It is common for patients to be in hospital for approximately two or three months.

Chronic neuropathies

There are a variety of chronic diseases which can cause peripheral neuropathy. These include carcinoma of most organs, diabetes mellitus, hypothyroidism, acromegaly, liver failure, leprosy, and some hereditary diseases such as Charcot–Marie–Tooth disease.

Factors other than disease can also cause peripheral neuropathy, including industrial substances (e.g. lead, organic solvents and organic phosphates) and certain drugs (e.g. phenytoin, isoniazid and vincristine).

Further reading

Bickerstaff, E.R. (1978) *Neurology,* 3rd edition. London: Hodder & Stoughton.

Myco, F. (1983) *Nursing Care of the Hemiplegic Stroke Patient* New York and London: Harper & Row.

Nursing 2 (1983) *Neurological Nursing* Volumes 15 and 16 (July and August).

Purchese, G. & Allan, D. (1984) *Neuromedical and Neurosurgical Nursing,* 2nd edition. London: Baillière Tindall.

Van Zwanonberg, D. & Adams, L.B.T. (1979) *Neurosurgical Nursing* London: Faber & Faber.

15
Endocrinological Nursing

The endocrine glands secrete chemical substances called hormones directly into the bloodstream. These hormones are then carried to other tissues of the body where they stimulate or depress metabolic processes. In this chapter the following endocrine glands will be considered:

pituitary
thyroid
parathyroids
pancreas
adrenals

Their positions in the body are shown in Figure 54.

THE PITUITARY GLAND

The pituitary gland lies in a hollow in the sphenoid bone at the base of the skull. It is stimulated by the hypothalamus of the brain. The hypothalamus regulates the amount of hormones secreted by the pituitary into the blood.

The pituitary gland consists of an anterior and a posterior lobe. *The anterior lobe* produces growth hormone (GH), thyroid stimulating hormone (TSH), adrenocorticotrophic hormone (ACTH), prolactin and the gonadotrophic hormones. *The posterior lobe* produces oxytocin and antidiuretic hormone (ADH, vasopressin).

Disorders of the pituitary gland

Dwarfism

Dwarfism is caused by a deficiency of growth hormone in early life. The person is normal in all respects except stature. Injection of human growth hormone will stimulate growth and enable the

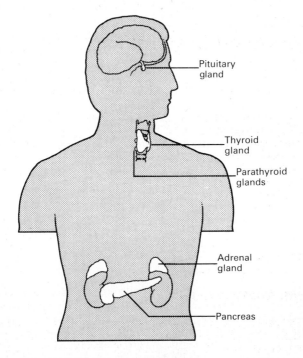

Figure 54. Position of the endocrine glands.

child to reach a normal height. The psychological effects of dwarfism are enormous; the child should be encouraged to participate in social activities which are in accordance with his age.

Gigantism

Gigantism is caused by hypersecretion of growth hormone in childhood. This is usually due to a tumour (adenoma) of the pituitary gland. If left untreated the individual can grow to 2–2.5 m (7–8 ft) tall. Pressure from the adenoma can cause headaches, vomiting and blindness. Treatment is the removal of the pituitary gland. Replacement of one or more of the hormones normally secreted by the gland may be necessary after surgery.

Acromegaly

Acromegaly is caused by hypersecretion of growth hormone in an adult, after fusion of the epiphyses of the long bone. Bone thickens, especially that of the hands, feet and skull. Facial disfiguration may occur and speech may be affected. Acromegaly is to due a tumour of the pituitary gland. Methods of treatment include:

Radioactive implants
Radiotherapy
Hypophysectomy (removal of the pituitary gland)
Cryosurgery (liquid nitrogen freezing)
Drugs (bromocriptine reduces the levels of growth hormone)

After treatment, replacement therapy with thyroxine, cortisone, oestrogen or testosterone may be necessary.

The patient with acromegaly may have become very embarrassed about his altered appearance and will therefore need much psychological support from the nurse.

Simmond's syndrome

Simmond's syndrome is atrophy or destruction of the anterior lobe of the pituitary gland. The causes are infarction resulting from postpartum haemorrhage, tumour, trauma, infection or surgical removal. Clinical features are weakness, weight loss, amenorrhoea, atrophy of the genital organs and loss of axillary and pubic hair.

Fludrocortisone, thyroxine and oestrogen or testosterone are used as replacement therapy.

Diabetes insipidus

Diabetes insipidus is characterized by the persistent excretion of excessive quantities of urine of low specific gravity and by constant thirst, and is due to undersecretion of antidiuretic hormone (ADH, vasopressin). Causes include damage to the posterior pituitary from tumour, surgery, trauma (e.g. fractured base of skull) or idiopathic malfunction.

Medical and nursing problems
Polyuria
— excessive quantities of urine (5–20 l)
— low specific gravity (1000–1004)

Dehydration
— thirst
— dry tongue
— inelastic skin
Electrolyte imbalance

Medical treatment
- Severe dehydration will be corrected immediately with intravenous fluids and electrolytes.
- A water deprivation test will be performed. Fluids are withheld for a specified period and, if diabetes insipidus is present, polyuria will persist.
- Replacement therapy is commenced by giving a synthetic vasopressin derivative (Pitressin) as a nasal spray or by intramuscular injection. This treatment must continue for life.
- Chlorpropamide or chlorothiazide may also be given as they help to reduce the polyuria.

Nursing intervention
- Fluid intake and output are recorded, together with the specific gravity of the urine.
- The patient will require frequent mouthwashes to keep the mouth clean and moist.
- Pressure area care is given two-hourly to prevent damage to the dry, inelastic skin.

THE THYROID GLAND

The thyroid gland is situated in the neck, in front of the trachea. It manufactures thyroid hormone (thyroxine) which is released into the bloodstream as required. Thyroid hormone controls the basal metabolic rate and is essential for normal mental and physical development and for normal function of the nervous system.

Production of thyroid hormone is controlled by the hypothalmus via the anterior pituitary gland.

Disorders of the thyroid gland

Hyperthyroidism (thyrotoxicosis)

Hyperthyroidism (over-secretion of thyroid hormone) causes an increase in the metabolic rate of the body. The cause is uncertain but may possibly be due to an antibody found in the blood.

Medical and nursing problems
Weight loss
— with good appetite
Excitability
— anxiety
— restlessness
— tremor
Increased heart rate
— arrhythmias
— cardiac enlargement
Exophthalmos (protrusion of the eyeballs)

Medical treatment
- Sedatives such as diazepam may be required to reduce excitability.
- Disturbances in cardiac rhythm may be controlled with propranolol.
- Specific treatment of hyperthyroidism may include antithyroid drugs, radioactive iodine therapy or partial thyroidectomy.
- Antithyroid drugs, e.g. carbimazole, interfere with the production of thyroid hormone. High doses are given initially, followed by a smaller maintenance dose. This form of therapy is more suitable for children and for pregnant women.
- Radioactive iodine therapy involves the oral administration of a radioactive isotope ^{131}I which destroys some of the thyroid cells. This treatment is not given to women who are still in the reproductive period of life. There is a risk of hypothyroidism after this form of treatment.
- Partial thyroidectomy is mostly used in cases where drug therapy has not controlled the condition. Iodine is given in the preoperative period to decrease the vascularity of the gland.

Nursing intervention
- The patient is helped to rest as much as possible.
- A high-protein, high-carbohydrate diet is given.
- Pulse and respiration rate are recorded at least six-hourly in order to detect signs of cardiac failure.

Conclusion
The results of treatment are excellent, but exophthalmos usually persists.

Hypothyroidism may occur as a result of treatment with radioactive iodine or surgery. Long-term treatment with thyroxine may be necessary.

Hypothyroidism (myxoedema)

Hypothyroidism is due to under-secretion of thyroxine. It may develop in adult life or may be congenital. It causes a decrease in the metabolic rate of the body. Causes include:

autoimmune disease
pituitary malfunction
radioactive iodine
surgery

Medical and nursing problems
Lethargy
Sensitivity to the cold
Slow pulse rate
Oedema around the eyes
Dry, brittle hair
Amenorrhoea
Anaemia
Constipation

Medical treatment
- Medical treatment is with thyroxine, administered daily for life. The dose is carefully adjusted to prevent symptoms of hypothyroidism.

Nursing intervention
- The patient will need continual encouragement as he tends to be slow and unmotivated.

- A diet which is high in roughage is given to prevent constipation.
- The patient is kept warm. Occasionally hypothermia occurs in an elderly person with hypothyroidism.

Conclusion

Hypothyroidism in children (cretinism), if not detected early, will lead to retardation of physical and mental development.

Results of treatment with thyroxine are excellent.

THE PARATHYROID GLANDS

The four parathyroid glands are situated in the neck behind the thyroid gland. These glands secrete parathyroid hormone (parathormone) which helps to regulate calcium and phosphate levels in the body.

Disorders of the parathyroid glands

Hyperparathyroidism

Hyperparathyroidism (over-activity of the parathyroid glands) may be primary or secondary.

Primary hyperparathyroidism is usually due to a benign tumour (an adenoma). The increase in parathyroid hormone causes calcium to be withdrawm from the bones and deposited in other parts of the body such as the renal and gastrointestinal tracts.

Secondary hyperparathyroidism is a compensatory enlargement of the parathyroid glands as a result of a reduction in the level of calcium in the blood which occurs in some diseases.

Medical and nursing problems

Lethargy

Anorexia

Muscle weakness

Polyuria

Abdominal pain

— due to calcium deposits in
gut wall and in kidneys

Loin pain

Bone pain

— due to calcium depletion
in bones

Fractures

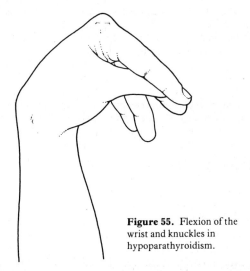

Figure 55. Flexion of the wrist and knuckles in hypoparathyroidism.

Medical treatment

- Treatment of primary hyperparathyroidism is surgical. Abnormal parathyroid tissue is removed.
- Secondary hyperparathyroidism is treated with oral vitamin D (dihydrotachysterol).

Nursing intervention

- The patient is encouraged to drink two-and-a-half litres of fluid each day to prevent formation of renal stones.
- A 24-hour urine collection is commenced for urinary calcium levels.

Hypoparathyroidism

Hypoparathyroidism (under-activity of the parathyroid glands) may result in tetany. Causes include:

idiopathic
accidental removal during surgery
injury
disease

Medical and nursing problems

Muscle twitching

Tingling sensations

Flexion of wrist and knuckles
(Figure 55)

Laryngeal spasm

Stridor

Obstruction

Convulsions

Depression

Psychosis

Medical and nursing intervention

- The emergency treatment for tetany is the intravenous administration of calcium gluconate.
- Maintenance therapy is with oral preparations of vitamin D (calciferol). The dosage is adjusted according to the plasma calcium levels.

THE PANCREAS

The endocrine functions of the pancreas include the secretion of insulin and glucagon.

Glucagon is produced by the alpha (α) cells of the islets of Langerhans. *Insulin* is produced by the beta (β) cells of the islets of Langerhans. Insulin and glucagon regulate the level of glucose in the blood.

Disorders of the pancreas

Pancreatitis and carcinoma of the pancreas are discussed in Chapter 9.

Diabetes mellitus

Diabetes mellitus is failure of the pancreas to secrete sufficent insulin to meet the body's requirements. This condition results in hyperglycaemia (high blood glucose levels). It is a chronic disease, and is common in Britain where it has a prevalence of over 2%. Eighty per cent of sufferers are over 50 years. Causes include:

Idiopathic

Familial tendency

Pancreatic disease, e.g. carcinoma, pancreatitis

Corticosteroid therapy

Abnormal levels of hormonal insulin antagonists, e.g. growth
hormone

Medical and nursing problems

Glycosuria
— often detected on routine urine testing

Polyuria
— due to increased osmotic pressure exerted by high concentration
of glucose

Polydipsia
— dehydration and thirst caused by polyuria

Weight loss ⎫
Lethargy ⎬ fat is broken down for energy production
Muscle wasting ⎭ instead of carbohydrates

Ketonuria ⎫ ketones are the breakdown
Smell of ketones on breath ⎬ products of fat metabolism

Vomiting
— due to ketoacidosis

Drowsiness

Coma
— death may occur

Medical investigation and treatment

- Blood is taken for glucose levels (normal fasting blood glucose
= 3.0–5.3 mmol/l).
- A glucose tolerance test is performed.
- There are three methods of treatment of diabetes mellitus: diet
alone, diet and oral hypoglycaemic drugs or diet and insulin.
- Diet involves restriction of carbohydrate in accordance with the
patient's weight, occupation, age and sex. An obese, elderly
patient will require only 4200–6720 kJ (1000–1600 kcal) daily
whereas a young active diabetic may need 7560–12600 kJ
(1800–3000 kcal) daily. The carbohydrate allowance is about
40% of this total.
- Oral hypoglycaemic drugs are given to mature-onset diabetics
who cannot be controlled on diet alone. These drugs include
tolbutamide, glibenclamide and chlorpropamide, which reduce
the release of glucose from the liver, and metformin and
phenformin, which increase the glucose uptake in the tissues.
Amount and timing of food intake should be regulated in order
that the blood sugar is kept as level as possible.

Hypoglycaemia may occur with hypoglycaemic drugs.

Insulin may be required in times of illness and stress.

- Subcutaneous insulin injections are always given to young diabetics. They require this form of treatment for the rest of their lives. During stabilization of the diabetes, the patient is encouraged to be as active as normal in order that the dosage of insulin can be matched to diet, physical activities and weight.

There are many types of insulin. Short-lasting insulins include soluble insulin and neutral insulin (Actrapid). Intermediate-acting insulins include semilente insulin zinc suspension (Semitard) isophane and Mixtard (isophane and neutral insulin). Long-acting insulins include lente insulin zinc suspension (Monotard). Diet is regulated as above.

Nursing intervention

- The urine is tested for glucose and ketones at least six-hourly. This test is performed before meals using a fresh specimen.
- Blood glucose can be measured by nursing staff using BM sticks or Dextrostix. An increasing number of electronic devices are available that can be used to measure capillary blood glucose levels.

Education of the diabetic

The new diabetic is supplied with a glass insulin syringe, disposable needles, syringe container and a urine testing kit. He is taught to test his own urine twice daily before meals. If it contains 2% glucose he should also test for ketones. Many diabetics are now also being taught to measure their own blood sugars.

The diabetic should learn how to draw up and inject insulin in various sites of the body (Figure 56). The most common sites are the thighs, abdomen and upper arms. The syringe is usually soaked in methylated spirits between use and it is important that the patient understands the need for cleanliness. Explanation should be given about the new standard 100 units/ml insulin (Figure 57). The diabetic can be taught to adjust his dose of insulin according to his needs, for example, more insulin with increased carbohydrate, less insulin with increased exercise. He should not miss a dose of insulin even if food intake is reduced.

The diabetic may be able to experience hypoglycaemia as part of his education. The onset of hypoglycaemia is rapid when the blood glucose level falls below 2 mmol/l. Sweating, tachycardia and

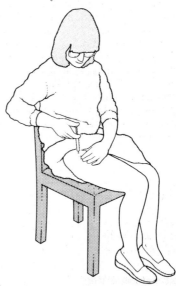

Figure 56.
Injection of insulin.

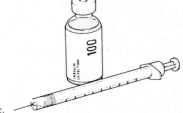

Figure 57.
An insulin syringe.

hunger occur quickly, followed by confusion and an alteration in consciousness. Treatment should be prompt. Milk and biscuits or glucose should be given. If consciousness is lost, intravenous 50% glucose or intramuscular glucagon is given. Failure to treat hypoglycaemia promptly may result in fits and coma. The patient should be told to always carry glucose with him. He should also have a card indicating that he is a diabetic.

Diabetics are vulnerable to infections of all kinds and these should be treated immediately. Insulin requirements will increase during an infection, in pregnancy and after surgery. The patient should be taught good skin care especially of the feet. They are advised to visit a chiropodist regularly.

Complications of diabetes

Vascular disorders
— myocardial infarction
— intermittent claudication
— gangrene (lower limbs)
Eye disorders
— retinopathy
— blindness
— cataracts
Renal disorders
— glomerulosclerosis
— renal failure

Infections
— carbuncles
— *Candida albicans*
— urinary tract infections
— pulmonary tuberculosis
Nerve disorders
— peripheral neuropathy
— muscle wasting

Diabetic ketoacidosis

This condition occurs in diabetics with severe hyperglycaemia when fat is broken down for energy production. Toxic acid products of fat metabolism (ketones) accumulate in the blood. Causes include:

New diabetic who has failed to seek medical help
Carelessness or ignorance
Illness or stress, which increases insulin requirements

Medical and nursing problems

Polyuria
Polydipsia
Dehydration
— low blood pressure
— tachycardia
— dry tongue
— inelastic skin
Vomiting
— due to ketoacidosis

Drowsiness
Coma
Deep respirations
Smell of acetone on breath

Medical investigation and treatment

- Blood is taken for glucose and electrolyte levels and arterial blood is taken to determine blood gases and pH.
- An intravenous infusion is commenced to correct the dehydration. Normal saline and 5% dextrose are given.
- Soluble or Actrapid insulin is given intramuscularly and intravenously. The dosage is calculated according to blood sugar estimations. Insulin may also be given via a constant infusion pump.
- Sodium bicarbonate is given intravenously to correct the acidosis.
- Potassium supplements are necessary to correct electrolyte imbalance.

Nursing intervention

- Care is required as for an unconscious patient (see page 32).
- Capillary blood sugar is estimated at least hourly using BM sticks or Dextrostix. Blood sugar should be maintained between 4 and 10 mmol/l.
- Urine is tested for glucose and ketones. A urinary catheter may be required.
- When the patient is awake he will commence a fluid diet containing measured amounts of carbohydrates and progress to a solid diet.

Conclusion

Diabetes is a disease of the prosperous, wealthy countries; mature-onset diabetes is liable to arise in people who eat too much and take too little exercise. Atherosclerosis is the most common cause of death in diabetics.

The diabetic should be encouraged to have a flexible lifestyle. Most occupations are open to diabetics. The British Diabetic Association offers support and education to its members.

Children and teenagers may need particular support as they may have difficulty in accepting their diabetes.

THE ADRENAL GLANDS

The two adrenal glands are situated on top of the kidneys. Each gland consists of an outer cortex and an inner medulla.

The adrenal cortex produces glucocorticoids (e.g. hydrocortisone), which are secreted in response to adrenocorticotrophic hormone (ACTH) from the pituitary gland, and mineralocorticoids (e.g. aldosterone). These hormones are important for the formation of glucose, the retention of salt and water, the manufacture of red blood cells, the maintenance of blood pressure and for the response of the body to stress. The cortex also produces androgens which influence the development of sexual characteristics.

The adrenal medulla secretes adrenaline and noradrenaline. These hormones prepare the body for physical exertion by increasing the blood pressure, heart rate, and the blood supply to the muscles, brain and lungs, and by releasing glycogen for conversion to glucose.

Disorders of the adrenal glands

Addison's disease

Addison's disease is chronic undersecretion of the hormones from the adrenal cortex. It is caused by atrophy or destruction by tuberculosis of both adrenal glands.

Medical and nursing problems

Low blood pressure
— dehydration due to
   sodium loss
Weakness
Giddiness and fainting
Diarrhoea
Vomiting
Weight loss
Dry, inelastic skin

Dry mouth
Sweating
— due to hypoglycaemia
Confusion
Skin pigmentation
Menstrual disturbances
Diminished response to
   stress, e.g. infection,
   injury

Medical investigation and treatment

- Acute adrenal failure is treated promptly with intravenous fluids and electrolytes.
- Dextrose 5% is given intravenously to raise the blood sugar.
- Hydrocortisone is given by intravenous injection.
- Long-term replacement of hormones with cortisol and fludrocortisone is required. The dosage is altered according to the patient's particular needs. More cortisol is necessary in times of stress, including minor illnesses. The patient is taught to adjust the dosage himself.
- A steroid card should be carried at all times. Treatment with steroids should never be stopped abruptly.

Nursing intervention

- The patient with acute adrenal failure should be nursed flat with the foot of the bed elevated to maintain blood pressure.
- Accurate fluid input and output charts are kept.
- Blood pressure is monitored carefully and the patient's level of consciousness is observed.
- Urine is tested for glucose.
- Reassurance is necessary as the patient will probably be frightened.
- Mouth care is given two-hourly in order to keep the mouth clean and moist.
- Pressure area care is required.

Cushing's syndrome

Cushing's syndrome is the result of oversecretion of hormones from the adrenal cortex. It is caused by hyperplasia of the adrenals or by a pituitary tumour producing excess ACTH. Administration of therapeutic corticosteroids also may produce symptoms of Cushing's syndrome.

Medical and nursing problems

Muscle wasting	Amenorrhoea
Glycosuria	Facial hair
— steroid-induced diabetes	Impotence
	Susceptibility to bruising

Obesity of the trunk   Purple striae
Moon face   Osteoporosis
Thin arms and legs   Fractures
Hypertension

Medical and nursing intervention
Adrenal hyperplasia is treated by a bilateral adrenalectomy. There
is a serious risk of an adrenal crisis associated with this operation.
Pituitary tumours are removed or irradiated. If the syndrome is
caused by therapeutic steroids, the dosage is adjusted.

Steroid-induced diabetes is treated with diet and hypoglycaemic
drugs or diet and insulin. The patient should be taught to test his
own urine.

Phaeochromocytoma

Phaeochromocytoma is a rare tumour of the adrenal medulla
which secretes excessive adrenaline and noradrenaline.
Hypertension, sweating, tachycardia and other symptoms of
increased metabolism occur.

Treatment is surgical removal of the tumour.

Further reading

British Diabetic Association (1972) *Diabetics Handbook* London: British
    Diabetic Association.
Nursing 2 (1983) *Hormones* Volumes 13 and 14 (May and June).
Oakley, W.G. et al (1978): *Diabetes and its Management,* 3rd edition.
    Oxford: Blackwell Scientific.

Index